Out of the Blues

Dealing with the Blues of Depression and Loneliness

Dr. Wayne Mack

Out of the Blues:
Dealing with the Blues of
Depression and Loneliness
by Dr. Wayne Mack

Scripture references are quoted from
The New American Standard Version of the Bible
and where noted,
The King James Version
and The New King James Version

Cover design by Melanie Schmidt

ISBN 1-885904-59-2

PRINTED IN THE UNITED STATES OF AMERICA
BY
FOCUS PUBLISHING
Bemidji, Minnesota

Introduction

When a Christian friend heard that I was writing a book discussing a biblical perspective on depression, she sent me a note to encourage me in this endeavor. The note indicated that she thought a book like this was very needed and relevant as she said, "Half the people I know are on Zoloft! Actually, I'm the happiest person I know!!"

Of course, I knew the subject was relevant because of my own counseling experience. During the more than thirty years I have been involved in the ministry of biblical counseling, I have been called upon to help people who are experiencing depression as much as for any other problem. Some have come acknowledging they were depressed; others who were depressed were calling it something else. In addition to what my counseling experience has taught me, I knew that a book like this was needed because of my research experience. In my research for presenting seminars on counseling depressed people, I discovered there are many books on the topic written by secular counselors, and there are numerous books in which Bible verses and biblical examples are sometimes superficially quoted. However, finding a book where solid exegesis of Scripture was practiced was almost an exercise in futility. So my research experience convinced me that a book presenting a distinctly biblical perspective on depression would be a valuable resource for counselors and individuals alike.

I don't claim to have written everything the Bible has to say about depression. God's Word is so exceedingly deep and broad that it would be impossible for any person to completely exhaust what the Bible has to say about any subject (Psalm 119:96).

Even so, I believe that my understanding of what Scripture has to say about depression is accurate as far as it goes. What I know from Scripture I know truly, but because of the depth and breadth of God's Word there is always more to learn. Therefore, while making no claim to complete comprehensiveness, it is my hope that this book about depression and its frequently attendant experience of loneliness accurately reflects Scriptural truth and therefore will help you to avoid or get out of the "blues".

In writing this book, I have attempted to present a biblical perspective on the nature, causes and solution to the problems of depression and loneliness. I have approached this task with the conviction that an all-knowing God has given us in His Word everything we need for living and for godliness and that the "everything we need" includes what we need to understand and defeat depression and loneliness.

In the first part of the book, I seek to define and describe depression biblically. In the second part of the book I deal with the development or dynamics of depression. In the third section, I present the biblical solution to the problem. The last chapter of the book explores the nature, causes and solution to the blues caused by loneliness. To make the material very practical, useful and applicatory, I have included study questions for each chapter. Some are review questions that will enable you to fix the truths of the chapter in your thinking. Some are thought and application questions that will encourage you to take the truths of the chapter out of the realm of theory and into daily life and practice.

Two of the unique features of this book are found in Chapters 7 and 8. Chapter 7 is titled "Questions and Answers about Depression". In this chapter I give my perspective on some of the questions I have been asked over the years. Chapter 8 is entitled, "Additional Notes for the Counselor". In this chapter I seek to give some pertinent directions for helping another person who is experiencing depression. The suggestions presented in this chapter are especially relevant for people who function as formal counselors, but they will also be useful for family members or friends, and even for depressed persons in biblically understanding and solving the problem of depression.

As you read on, I urge you to follow two biblical examples. Follow the example of the Bereans as described in Acts 17:11: They searched the Scriptures to make sure that what Paul was telling them was biblically accurate. I urge you to do the same with what I have written in this book. Likewise, I urge you to follow Paul's exhortation to the Thessalonians in 1 Thessalonians 5:21. I challenge you to examine everything I write carefully; compare it to what the Scriptures say, and hold fast to that which is good (that which is really biblical). Don't accept what I write because I write it. Accept what is written in this book only if it is an accurate portrayal of what God says in His Word. You don't need more theories of finite and fallible men about depression. You need the wisdom of a God who knows everything about everything, including depression, and you will find that wisdom in Scripture. And, to the extent that what I have written is an accurate reflection of Scripture you will find God's wisdom about depression in this book as well.

I thank God for the privilege of studying and ministering His Word, and I thank you for allowing me to communicate to you some important concepts I have learned from His Word. I also want to thank Janet Dudek, who helped me with the editing and shaping of the material in this book. Without her expertise and faithful labors, this book would not have seen the light of day for a long time.

My desire is that our great all-wise and loving God would make your reading and study of this book a fruitful experience in your own personal life and in your ministry to others as well.

Dr. Wayne Mack

Table of Contents

                                                                     Page

Introduction

1.	What's it Like to be Depressed?	1
2.	What's it Like to be **REALLY** Depressed?	15
3.	Why Do People Get Depressed?	33
4.	Getting Out of the Blues: Biblical Principles	61
5.	Getting Out of the Blues: Biblical Examples	81
6.	Loneliness or Lonely-less?	95
7.	Questions and Answers about Depression	111
8.	Additional Notes for the Counselor	129

Chapter 1
What's it Like to be Depressed?
Defining and Describing the Problem

Concerned about his very depressed wife, a man made an appointment with a psychiatrist. When they entered the office, the doctor began by asking the wife a few questions. As they talked, the doctor got up and sat down right beside the woman. The woman seemed surprised, but pleased. As they continued to talk, the doctor put his arm around the woman and smiled into her face. She smiled back. A moment later, he gave her a squeeze on the shoulders, leaned over, and planted a kiss on her cheek. By that time, the woman was beaming.

The psychiatrist then got up, returned to his chair, and said to the woman's husband, "Did you see how your wife's mood changed when I sat down beside her, smiled at her, hugged her, and gave her a kiss on the cheek?" "Yes," the man replied. "Well," continued the psychiatrist, "That's the kind of treatment she needs, and she needs it at least three times a week." "Okay," agreed the husband, "If that's what you think she needs, then I'll bring her here every Tuesday and Thursday, but I can't bring her on Saturday because that's my golf day."

While this story may be fictitious, the problem the woman was experiencing is not. Depression is a common and very serious problem. Indeed, her problem was not going to be solved by someone simply showing her a little attention three times a week, though it would not have hurt. And while this story may be amusing, the problem of depression is far from humorous. It devastates and cripples the lives it infects, wrecks marriages and other relationships, and–in the case of believers–damages faith. It is not to be taken lightly.

THE COMMONALITY OF DEPRESSION

I have heard it said by some "mental health experts" that depression is the common cold of mental ailments. In other words, depression is such a common human experience that nearly every person–regardless of their background–will experience it to some degree or another during their lifetime. They support their claims with surveys indicating that between seven and fifteen percent of the general population is suffering from depression at any given time. Other studies show that the incidence of depression is even higher.

Whatever the high end may be, the lower numbers–if correct–do represent a significant problem. In my experience, I found that depression is truly a democratic disorder, affecting people of all race, economic status, gender, age, and educational background. I have counseled young children who were depressed; one of them was only six years old when he attempted suicide. I have worked with teenagers who were depressed; some were failing in many areas of their lives, while others were doing well in school, had positions of leadership, were considered attractive and talented, and seemed to have great potential.

Though I agree with the "experts" in little else involving depression, I do agree with their assessment of the commonality of depression. As I write this book, I am convinced I am addressing a problem that nearly all of my readers have, or will struggle with, at some point. It is hard for me to imagine that there is anyone who will not be tempted to become depressed during his or her lifetime. And for those of us who are not currently struggling with this problem, I would guess that most of us know someone who is.

In 1968, I experienced a time of deep depression myself. By the grace of God, I was able to overcome that depression through biblical counseling. Therefore, the truths I am going to share in this book I share for both pastoral and personal reasons. I believe the Bible teaches these truths. I have seen them work in the lives of people struggling with depression, and God has used them in my own life to help me overcome depression.

Since depression is so common, it is important that *all* believers know how to deal with it as God intended. Whether for our own benefit or for the benefit of others we may be able to help, it is crucial that we understand what *God's solution* to this problem is. In order to do that, we will begin our study by looking at what God's perspective is–as revealed to us in Scripture–on what depression is and how it develops. In later chapters, we will study some biblical strategies for resolving the problem itself.

A NECESSARY CLARIFICATION

Before we continue, I would like to clarify the fact that the kind of depression we will be discussing in this book is depression that is *not* directly caused by some malfunction or physical disease. In a minority of cases, feelings of depression may be the byproduct of a physical illness or disorder. *The Christian Counselor's Medical Desk Reference*[1] lists many physical problems that may cause this: Alzheimer's disease, Parkinson's disease, and certain cancers, among others. In these cases, it is not appropriate for the condition to be called depression, according to Dr. Robert Smith and other Christian physicians. Instead, it should be described according to whatever physical ailment the person is experiencing. If there is any suspicion that a physical ailment may be causing the down mood, a thorough and appropriate physical exam should be sought from a medical doctor.

Where physical exams have demonstrated the presence of some physical ailment, treatment with legitimate remedies will constitute a large part of the solution to the feelings of depression. That said, the experts I have talked to agree that this applies to less than twenty percent of people experiencing down moods.[2] (Much more about the physical aspects of some down moods may be found in *The Christian Counselor's Medical Desk Reference* by Dr. Robert Smith that is published by Timeless Texts. Later in this book we will also briefly suggest some questions that may help you to discern whether there may be a physical component to the depressive mood.)

Additionally, we will *not* be discussing the kind of depression caused by the influence of certain drugs–legal or illegal–on the brain. Again, in some cases, feelings of depression can result from physical changes caused by certain drugs. In our discussion of depression, it is important to keep in mind that we are not directly addressing any kind of depression that is physically or biologically induced. Though the truths presented will certainly have some application in these instances, they are not primarily directed towards such types of depression.

DEPRESSION: A CATCHALL TERM

The word "depression" is really a broad term that is used to describe quite a variety of emotional experiences. It includes feelings such as sadness, sorrow, heavy-heartedness, disappointment, discouragement, humiliation, dejection, gloom, disillusionment, demoralization, despondency, despair, or even just a "case of the blues." In diagram form, the word depression is used to describe many of the following experiences:

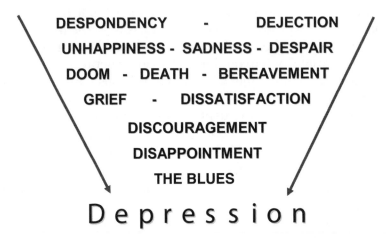

DESPONDENCY - DEJECTION

UNHAPPINESS - SADNESS - DESPAIR

DOOM - DEATH - BEREAVEMENT

GRIEF - DISSATISFACTION

DISCOURAGEMENT

DISAPPOINTMENT

THE BLUES

D e p r e s s i o n

For our purposes, we will separate the experience termed "depression" into three categories: mild depression; moderate depression; and severe depression.

CATEGORY 1
MILD DEPRESSION: AN INEVITABLE RESPONSE

Everyone experiences a "case of the blues" from time to time. Some people will say that they are "depressed" when they feel a bit discouraged, disappointed, or sad about something. In other words, they are not as content or happy as they usually are and they recognize that something is amiss.

Everyone suffers disappointment and discouragement at one time or another. A pastor friend of mine told me once that he experiences this weekly. He explained that, for him, Sunday is the highpoint of his week. It is the culmination of a week's work, a day in which he meets with and leads God's people in worship, and the day in which he has the high and holy privilege of preaching the Word of God. That one day each week consumes much of his physical, emotional, and spiritual energy.

Since Sunday is such a big day, one might expect that Monday would naturally be a bit of a letdown from his mountaintop on Sunday. He shared with me that, because he always feels a little down on Mondays, he stopped taking it as his day off. Instead of spending his day off feeling blue, he works through the day and is able to enjoy a day off later in the week, after his temporary gloom has passed. He recognized a situation that could potentially bring down his mood and took steps to avoid it.

What my friend experienced every Monday was a "case of the blues," or *mild depression*. This kind of depression might be better termed "discouragement" or "disappointment." It is a very common experience that comes and goes with the ups and downs of daily life. In fact, the Bible says that even Jesus, who was perfect, was "a man of sorrows and acquainted with grief" (Isaiah 53:3).

According to the gospel accounts, Jesus as a perfect man experienced sorrow, weariness, discouragement and disappointment just as we do. He was, as the Scripture indicates, tempted in all points as we are (Hebrews 2:17, 18 and 4:15). However, though He was grieved over the effects of sin in the lives of others and in the world, he never allowed Himself to be controlled by these feelings. Christ *always* fulfilled his responsibilities in spite of His circumstances: "... for I always do the things that are pleasing to Him" (John 8:29).

His actions following the death of John the Baptist are a good example of this. In Matthew 14, Herod had John the Baptist beheaded. After burying John, his disciples went and told Jesus. "When Jesus heard it, *He departed from there by boat to a deserted place by Himself.* But when the multitudes heard it, they followed Him on foot from the cities" (14:13). Jesus wanted time alone after receiving this difficult news, but was prevented from doing so because the crowds followed Him. "And when Jesus went out He saw a great multitude; and *He was moved with compassion for them, and healed their sick*" (14:14, emphasis added). Responsibility to His ministry immediately took precedence over His desire for time alone.

In John 6, we find another example of a time when Christ experienced disappointment. This passage contains a powerful message from Jesus described by some as containing a "difficult statement" that was hard to accept (John 6:60). His central point in this message was the teaching that He was the "bread" of Heaven. Jesus said, "I am the bread of life; he who comes to Me will not hunger, and he who believes in Me will never thirst" (6:35).

Though this statement may seem simple enough on the surface, his listeners apparently recognized that Christ was making some astounding assertions about Himself with these words. He used bread as an illustration because everyone would have been very familiar with it. If we understand what His listeners would have known about bread, then we can understand the impact of Christ's teaching here. James M. Boice pointed out the four significant assertions of Christ in this statement:[3]

First, *bread is necessary for life*. In Christ's time, bread was even more essential than it is today because it was often the sole staple of their diet. Without bread, men died. Second, *bread is suited for everyone*. In other words, bread is something that almost every person in the world can and does eat. Third, *bread must be eaten daily*. It is not enough to eat a meal on Sunday and expect it to last for the rest of the week. Fourth, *bread produces growth*. Without adequate nutrition, the body does not develop properly.

Considering that all of Christ's listeners would have known and understood these truths about bread, Christ's claim to be the "bread of life" was astounding indeed. In other words, Christ claimed to be the source of life, and by extension, implied that those without Him would die. Further, He claimed to be suited for everyone; able to meet the needs of all people whether rich or poor, young or old, Jew or Gentile.

Christ also claimed to be a necessary part of their everyday lives–requiring an on-going relationship–and a necessary source of adequate sustenance for growth. He taught that without a daily sufficient measure of Himself, the Word (John 1:1), people would become spiritually weak and ineffective for ministry. (Adapted from Boice, *Bible Studies*, John 6:28-37, pp. 12-15).[4]

In this "simple" statement that Christ made, many of His listeners recognized His claim to absolute uniqueness. Christ was saying that He was not just *some* bread; He was *the* bread *of life*. This was indeed a very difficult statement to hear and accept, and some of the people listening to Him decided that they had heard enough. "As a result of this, many of His disciples withdrew and were not walking with Him anymore" (John 6:66).

Jesus then turned to the disciples that remained (the twelve) and asked, "You do not want to go away also, do you?"(6:67). The question served as both a challenge to those disciples who stayed and as an expression of His concern about the response of those who had left. Though it did not affect His ministry, Jesus must have felt some disappointment at seeing so many of His followers leave at that time.

John 11 records yet another occasion of disappointment and sorrow for our Lord Jesus Christ. While ministering in another place, Jesus was told that his friend Lazarus, who lived in Bethany, was very sick. Jesus and his companions traveled to Bethany a few days later to see Lazarus, who had by that time died. When they arrived, Martha met Jesus with these words: "Lord, if You had been here, my brother would not have died" (John 11:21). Jesus answered by telling her that her brother would live again because He, Jesus, was the Resurrection and the Life (23-25).

After Martha left, Jesus encountered Mary, who immediately said the very same words that Martha had just spoken to Him. As she said them, however, Mary fell at Jesus' feet and wept (32-33). This time, His response was different. "When Jesus therefore saw her weeping…He was deeply moved in spirit and was troubled" (33). Why did Jesus weep at this time and not before? It was not because Lazarus was dead; Jesus knew already that he was dead and that He was going to raise Lazarus from the dead. He told His disciples that before they left for Bethany (6-15).

No, Jesus wept because He was "deeply moved in spirit" by the grief of Mary and the others. He sympathized with their sorrow. Though Jesus was always without sin, He expressed genuine sorrow over the difficulties and distresses of life. We, who are far from perfect, likewise experience discouragement and disappointment in this far from perfect world. Christ always knew the joy of the Lord to the fullest extent, but His emotions fluctuated to some degree with His external circumstances, just as ours do.

Some day in Heaven we also will know fullness of joy as Christ did, "In Your presence is fullness of joy; in Your right hand there are pleasures forever" (Psalm 16:11b). Sometimes, by God's grace, we get a taste of that even on earth. "These things I have spoken to you so that My joy may be in you, and *that your joy may be made full*" (John 15:11). However, our joy on this earth will always be mingled with sorrow, as evidenced by Paul's experience. After describing the immense difficulties that he faced in his ministry, he wrote, "But in everything commending ourselves as servants of God…*as sorrowful yet always rejoicing"* (2 Corinthians 6:4, 10).

I know of some Christians who think it is wrong for believers to ever be disappointed or sad. "Christians," they say, "should always be smiling." They believe that this is what Paul taught in Philippians 4:4 when He commanded us to "rejoice in the Lord always." It seems to me that this cannot be what Paul meant, as the Scripture teaches in many places that joy and sorrow can legitimately exist in our hearts at the same time.

For example, Ecclesiastes 3:4 says that there is "a time to weep and a time to laugh." The apostle Peter, after describing some of the blessings we have as believers, said, "In this you *greatly rejoice,* even though now for a little while, if necessary, you have been *distressed by various trials"* (1 Peter 1:6). His teaching makes it clear that it is *necessary* for us to feel the distress of trials, even as we greatly rejoice in our blessings in Christ. And the apostle Paul wrote, "But we do not want you to be uninformed brethren, about those who are asleep, *so that you will not grieve as do the rest who have no hope"* (1 Thessalonians 4:13, emphasis added).

The Scripture reveals that as long as we do not lose hope, there is nothing wrong with feeling the emotional down of sad and difficult events in our lives. In 1 Thessalonians, Paul was not teaching that, when difficult things happen (like the death of a loved one), we should not grieve. He was teaching that we should not grieve *and have no hope.* In other words, we should never forget the hope that we have in the coming of Christ Jesus and the promised resurrection of the dead. That is our *joy* in the midst of our *sorrow.*

CATEGORY 2
MODERATE DEPRESSION: THE WRONG RESPONSE

An experience of mild depression–sorrow, heaviness, discouragement or disappointment–is to be expected in the lives of all believers at various times. The nature of our response to this experience, however, is what determines the outcome and is what *should* set us apart from the unbelieving world around us. There are two basic responses to mild depression:

1. The Wrong Response: acknowledgement and
    submission to feelings

2. The Right Response: acknowledgement, but not submission to feelings

When some people experience mild depression, they acknowledge the reality of their feelings, but refuse to allow themselves to be controlled by them. In obedience to God's Word, they choose to "set their minds on things above, not on earthly things" (Colossians 3:2) and to "meditate on things that are good, pure, lovely, true, excellent, and praiseworthy" (Philippians 4:8). As they do this, they find that the light of God's Word burns away the cloud of heaviness in their hearts.

Other people pay far too much attention to their feelings, choosing to focus on them rather than on God. While focusing *on God* reduces the intensity of painful emotions, focusing *on emotions* has the opposite effect. Feelings of depression are magnified by the attention they receive and begin to control thoughts and actions. People who do this are ruled by their spirits, neglect biblical responsibilities, lose hope, and find that they get less and less satisfaction from spiritual things.

As their focus remains on their circumstances and the feelings generated by those circumstances, these people often find that they begin to cry easily, become easily annoyed, experience longer periods of sadness, and have difficulty performing the normal activities of life. Their minds are set on the negative aspects of their life–earthly things–rather than on God's promises, purposes, and power–things above. What started as mild depression becomes *moderate depression*.

Biblical Examples of Moderate Depression

Before we consider some biblical examples, it is necessary for me to say this about my use of examples from Scripture. I will be using events and people from the Bible as illustrations of moderate depression. By this I mean that I am using these accounts in Scripture for the purpose of gleaning insight on this subject, though I am in no way implying that these passages were written in the Scripture for the primary purpose of teaching on the subject of depression. God's primary purpose for including these passages, in most cases, was something else entirely.

Asaph

The first example is that of Asaph, the writer of Psalm 73. In this psalm, Asaph described what was happening in his life in this way:

> But as for me, my feet came close to stumbling, my steps had almost slipped. For I was envious of the arrogant as I saw the prosperity of the wicked...(vs. 2,3).

> Surely in vain I have kept my heart pure and washed my hands in innocence; for I have been stricken all day long and chastened every morning...(vs. 13-14).

> When I pondered to understand this, it was troublesome in my sight...(v. 6). When my heart was embittered and I was pierced within, Then I was senseless and ignorant; I was like a beast before You (vs. 21-22).

With these words, Asaph indicated that he was close to renouncing his faith. He admitted to being envious of others, discouraged, resentful, troubled, perplexed, full of self-pity, and generally miserable. He was thinking, feeling, and acting wrongly and his words imply that this had been going on for some time. Asaph was clearly not experiencing a simple case of the blues, or mild depression; his experience was much too deep and seemingly permanent for that.

Yet his depression was not of the most severe type because it is apparent from the rest of the Psalm that he never gave up entirely. He wrote that he "came *close* to stumbling" and his "steps...*almost* slipped." He was troubled, confused, and close to losing his self-control, but he was never completely devastated, utterly disillusioned, or totally consumed by his self-absorption. Verse 15 makes it clear that he still retained some control over himself, and this helped him to remember some important things about God (which we will look at later) that eventually lifted his depression.

Jeremiah

The great prophet Jeremiah also experienced moderate depression at least once during his time of ministry. In the book of Lamentations, he used metaphorical language to describe his emotional experience. He wrote of being in black darkness, being broken, having gall and travail, being chained, being hemmed in and trapped, being filled with bitterness, being far off from peace, being weary and fatigued, and crying and being shut out (Lamentations 3:1-20).

Again, this was clearly not a mild depression. Jeremiah was experiencing serious emotional turmoil and darkness, and yet his depression never became severe because he still had hope. He was still able to redirect his thoughts to the greatness of God and the greatness of His promises. In fact, his thoughts in this chapter fluctuate back and forth between discouraging and encouraging things. Though he was knocked down and damaged for a period of time–both physically and emotionally–and probably not serving the Lord as joyfully as he could or should have, he was not ready to give up entirely (Lamentations 3:21-66).

A Psalmist

"Why are you in despair, O my soul? And why have you become disturbed within me?" (Psalms 42 and 43). The writer of these two Psalms asked this question three times. He followed these questions with some indication of his depressed condition:

> My tears have been my food day and night,
> While they say to me all day long, "Where is your God?"
> O my God, my soul is in despair within me"…
> Why do I go mourning because of the oppression
> of the enemy?" (42:3, 6, 9b)

This man seems to be sorrowing over a lost sense of the presence of God in his life. "My soul thirsts for God, for the living God; when shall I come and appear before God?" (Psalm 42:2). He appears to be distraught by the mocking and oppression of his enemies (42:9-10) and his inability to lead God's people in worship as he formerly had (42:4). The constancy and seriousness of his trials was almost more than he could bear. "Deep calls to deep at the sound of Your waterfalls; all Your breakers and Your waves have rolled over me" (42:7).

Once again, however, we see that this man is not utterly cast down despite his present misery. He was most certainly struggling with moderate depression, but he did not give up entirely. He still had faith and hope in God as he wrote, "Hope in God, for I shall yet praise Him, the help of my countenance and my God" (42:11). He still found comfort in God's Word and believed that God would eventually deliver him, "O send out Your light and Your truth, let them lead me; let them bring me to Your holy hill" (43:3).

SUMMARY

Thus far, we have looked at the characteristics of mild and moderate depression and considered some biblical examples of each. In the next chapter, we will take a close look at the nature of severe depression and some people in the Bible who experienced it. This is all part of the first step in dealing with the problem of depression—or any other problem—and that is recognition. We are seeking to accurately define this problem because an accurate diagnosis is the first step to a successful cure. And now to make this chapter as useful as possible, I encourage you to spend some time answering the following discussion and application questions:

QUESTIONS FOR DISCUSSION AND APPLICATION:

1. How common is the problem of depression in society?

2. What is meant by the statement that depression is a truly "democratic" disorder?

3. What are the three categories of depression?

4. Why is the word "depression" described as a "catchall term"?

5. What biblical examples were given of the first category of depression?

6. What are some of the symptoms of this kind of depression?

7. What reasons were given to support the idea that there is nothing wrong with a Christian experiencing sorrow?

8. What biblical examples were given of the second category of depression?

9. What are some of the symptoms of this kind of depression?

Chapter 2
What's it Like to be
<u>REALLY</u> Depressed?

Depression is a serious problem that has been a common part of human experience from ancient times. While mild depression may last for a few hours or days, moderate depression goes deeper and generally lasts much longer. In the last chapter, we looked at the moderate depression of Asaph, Jeremiah, and a psalmist. We saw that all three were characterized by strong, distressing emotions, but in all three cases, the men who experienced this kind of depression never completely lost hope (as we will see more clearly in Chapter 5). They were still able to redirect their thoughts toward God and in so doing, avoided falling into utter despair. In other words, they were able to deal with their moderate depression before it became *severe depression*.

CATEGORY 3
SEVERE DEPRESSION

There is a kind of depression that goes deeper and is more serious than the moderate depression illustrated by Asaph, Jeremiah, and the psalmist. Severe depression is distinguished from moderate depression by the presence of utter hopelessness. A person experiencing moderate depression is most definitely down, but a severely depressed person is down *and out*. It is not just *difficult* for this person to keep going. The severely depressed person thinks it is *impossible* to keep going.

As we continue in this study, the definition of severe depression that we will use is this: It is a permanent spirit of heaviness or gloom that affects, controls, and dominates every area of a person's life.

A Biblical Description of Severe Depression

In John 16:6, Jesus described the experience of a severely depressed person as He told His disciples, "But because I have said these things to you, *sorrow has filled your heart*." The word "filled" indicates that there was room for *nothing else*, just as a cup that has been filled with water has room for no more liquid. When a person is severely depressed, their depression fills every aspect and facet of their life.

This is what happened to the disciples after Christ's death. They responded by just giving up. They ran to the upper room, locked the doors, and stayed there not knowing what to do. Sorrow had indeed "filled [their] hearts" and it caused them to abdicate their responsibilities and shut out the rest of the world for a time. They became severely depressed because they allowed their fear and disappointment to overpower and defeat them–they were ruled by their feelings.

David–Psalm 32

David's words in Psalm 32 are a good illustration of what happens to a severely depressed person because they reveal the great emotional and physical distress that he was experiencing at the time. Verses 3 and 4 describe his misery: "When I kept silent about my sin, my body wasted away through my groaning all day long. For day and night Your hand was heavy upon me; my vitality was drained away as with the fever heat of summer."

Notice first how David described himself. He said that his "body wasted away." He may have stopped eating, as the loss of one's appetite is a common experience among severely depressed people. As a result, these people often experience significant weight loss. They also experience physical deterioration due to the suppression of the immune system that accompanies any deep emotional distress.

David continued, "...through my groaning all day long." While no one feels like turning cartwheels every minute of their day, the spirit of heaviness that David described here is far more serious than the emotional ups and downs of a normal day or week. Most people, even on a "bad day," are able to continue with their normal activities and usually find that after a time, whatever gloom they may have started the day or week with eventually disappears.

A severely depressed person, however, wakes up feeling down and may or may not be even able to get out of bed, get dressed, or eat breakfast. The seemingly small and easy tasks of everyday life seem impossible for them to accomplish, requiring (in their minds) far more energy than they think they are capable of generating. The only task they find easy is that of continuing to dwell on their misery. This physical paralysis continues all day long, rendering them virtually useless to themselves or anyone else.

David went on, "For day and night Your hand was heavy upon me..." These words indicate that he felt as if he was under the burden of a great weight. Severely depressed people often express a feeling of tremendous weight on their shoulders, as if someone was constantly pressing down on them. They literally feel as if they are "carrying the weight of the world on their shoulders," and often walk around slowly and somewhat bent over.

He continued, "...my vitality was drained away as with the fever heat of summer." Anyone who has toiled for long hours under a hot summer sun knows what it feels like to have one's strength drained away by that intense heat. As a farmer's son, I worked many long hours under a hot summer sun. We used old-fashioned tools to cut and bind wheat straw, and then we stacked them in piles for drying. Later, the piles were brought into the barn to be threshed. Threshing was done in the hottest part of the summer and meant working in a constant cloud of dust, most of which seemed to cling to the sweat on our bodies. By the end of the day, we were physically wiped out; dusty, hot, tired, and hungry.

A severely depressed person feels that kind of fatigue–the kind of fatigue that one feels after an exhausting day of physical labor. He or she is literally "running on empty" and that is why even the smallest of tasks seems impossible to accomplish. When a person judges themselves to be incapable of even dressing or eating, then fellowshipping with the Lord in prayer and Bible study or going to church becomes, for them, out of the question. The weight of their emotional burden renders them too physically wasted to do *anything*.

David–Psalm 38

An equally vivid description of severe depression is found in Psalm 38, in which David wrote, "There is no soundness in my flesh... there is no health in my bones..." (38:3). His words indicate that he was experiencing some amount of physical pain and a great amount of physical weakness. As we just noted, this is often the case for a severely depressed person.

Later in this Psalm, David said, "I am bent over and greatly bowed down; I go mourning all day long. For my loins are filled with burning, and there is no soundness in my flesh. I am benumbed and badly crushed; I groan because of the agitation of my heart" (38:6-8). Again, we see the images of a great burden; a crushing weight, misery, groaning, and physical pain that is plaguing him.

He also described himself as "mourning all day long." Severely depressed people often find themselves weeping uncontrollably over seemingly small things and sometimes for long periods of time. In my experience as a biblical counselor, I have worked with both women and men who were severely depressed and who cried easily. While women often break into tears for various reasons—some because of depression and some for other reasons—it is rather unusual for a man to break into tears during a counseling session.

That said, it has happened several times that a man has wept uncontrollably in my office. In almost every instance this has occurred, the man I was counseling was suffering from severe depression. I find that though they are almost powerless to stop themselves from doing it, they are often embarrassed by their own tears because of the social stigma in our society of men crying. Because of this stigma, a man's uncontrollable weeping is often a sign of deep emotional torment. David suffered that kind of depression at one time.

Elijah

The prophet Elijah was indisputably one of the godliest men who ever lived and was used powerfully by the Lord. Jesus confirmed this when He referred to John the Baptist as the greatest man who had ever lived (Matthew 11:11). Prior to this, the angel of the Lord who spoke to Zacharias, John's father, said that John the Baptist would perform his ministry "in the spirit and power of Elijah" (Luke 1:17). Later, when Jesus experienced the transfiguration, Elijah was one of the two believers from Old Testament times who appeared and spoke with Him (Matthew 17:1-3).

Considering these things, Elijah may rightly be regarded as a spiritual giant. Yet the Bible indicates that there was an extended period of time in Elijah's life when he experienced what can only be called a severe depression. The events leading up to this point in his life are recorded in 1 Kings 17 and 18, and include a mixture of both exciting and frustrating experiences.

While wicked people, such as King Ahab and Queen Jezebel, displayed their depravity, debauchery, rebellion, and brutality, God displayed His power, faithfulness, provision, and protection to Elijah. The last event before Elijah's depression takes hold was the calling down of fire from Heaven to burn up his water-soaked sacrifice. Following this display of God's power, the prophets of Baal–450 men– were killed and the famine on the land was ended with a heavy rain. Then Elijah learned that Queen Jezebel had sworn a vow to her gods to kill him. In 1 Kings 19:3-10, the Bible describes Elijah's response to this last event:

> And he was afraid and arose and ran for his life and came to Beersheba, ... and left his servant there. But he himself went a day's journey into the wilderness, and came and sat down under a juniper tree; and he requested for himself that he might die, and said, "It is enough; now, O Lord, take my life...." He lay down and slept under a juniper tree; and behold, there was an angel touching him, and he said to him, "Arise and eat." ...So he arose and ate and drank, and went in the strength of that food forty days and forty nights to Horeb... Then he came there to a cave and lodged there; and behold, the word of the Lord came to him, and He said to him, "What are you doing here, Elijah?" He said, "I have been very zealous for the Lord, the God of hosts; for the sons of Israel have forsaken Your covenant, torn down Your altars and killed Your prophets with the sword. And I alone am left; and they seek my life, to take it away."

F. W. Krummacher commented on these verses: "In this instance, Elijah's faith appears to have failed him. The very words of the sacred narrative seem to give us a significant hint respecting the state of his mind at this period." Krummacher went on to note that Elijah's focus was not on "God's promises, aid, power and faithfulness" at that point in his life, but rather on his circumstances. He was obsessed with thoughts about:

> "...the infuriated Jezebel threatening his life, and all the horrors of a cruel death. Instead of soaring above these on eagle's wings, and looking down upon them with sublime composure, as on former occasions,

the pressures of human terror seem to have been too strong for his mind, especially as backed by the disappointment of his hopes on Israel's account. So, "he arose and went for his life;" or, as others have rendered it, "he arose and went whither he would;" which serves further to intimate the obscurity of his course and the uncertainty of his steps. He had, at this time, no express Divine direction as to whether he should go. Hitherto, his Lord had always marked out his way for him distinctly, but not so now.

"...He went forth into the wide world in uncertainty, distracted by doubts, and unaccompanied by the consoling consciousness that he was taking this road for God.

"...his spirit was too afflicted for common society. Even the company of his faithful servant was burdensome to him. ...he went alone into the solitary wilderness, into the very heart of it, a whole day's journey, until the sun went down. He then threw himself upon the heath under a juniper tree, and sank down under the load of his melancholy thoughts.

"Thick darkness hung over the prophet's soul... Perplexed with regard to his vocation–nay, even with respect to God and his government–his soul lies in the midst of a thousand doubts and distressing thoughts. It seems tossed on a sea of troubles, without bottom or shore; and there appears but one step between him and utter despair.

"There he sits, like an exile in the midst of fearful solitude, as if cast out by God and the world, with his eyes fixed; full of gloomy and painful thoughts. ...He is heartily weary of painful conflicts and fruitless labors; his soul longs for rest. 'It is enough, O Lord! Take my life...' Elijah sat under his juniper tree and thought in his despondency that he was unable any longer to bear the burden of life. ... 'Why should I remain any longer in this land of travail? My existence is useless. It is enough; now, O Lord, take away my life.'[5]

Elijah was most certainly experiencing severe depression, and in counseling people with severe depression, I have come to see great similarity in their experiences and the experience of Elijah at that point in his life.

2 Corinthians 4:8-9 and Severe Depression

In 2 Corinthians 4:8-9, Paul made a statement that helps to explain the nature of severe depression. He wrote, "We are afflicted in every way, *but not crushed*, perplexed, *but not despairing*; persecuted, *but not forsaken*, struck down, *but not destroyed.*" Though Paul was describing how he and his companions were living in obedience to God, what he says was *not* happening to them is a good description of what *does* happen to someone who is severely depressed.

First, we learn that Paul and his companions have been "afflicted in every way." In other words, they have seen it all. There is nothing they have not suffered or been subjected to, save death. But Paul said that though they were afflicted in every way, they were "*not crushed.*" Afflictions may cause a few cracks here and there (as my wife says, "that's how the Light gets in"), but Christians do not have to ever be crushed. People who are experiencing severe depression have allowed their circumstances to crush them.

Paul also wrote, "*We are perplexed*, but not despairing," meaning that they experienced some confusion during their ministry. They did not always understand what God was doing or why He was doing it. Despite their confusion, however, they were "not despairing." The Greek word *exaporeomai*, translated "despairing," means "to be utterly at a loss." Paul was saying that though they had no answers, they never stopped believing that God did. Not understanding our circumstances–not seeing a way through the darkness to the other side–can lead to depression if a believer either forgets or does not truly believe that God is always in control. Severely depressed people may say they believe in God's control over their life and circumstances, but they do not really believe it. Paul remembered and firmly believed that God was in control.

Next, Paul wrote that they were "*persecuted*, but not forsaken." In using the word "persecuted," Paul indicated they were not merely being ignored or disregarded by people; Paul and his companions were being actively sought out for abuse and injury. They had enemies who were determined to do them harm. In spite of this, however, they never felt abandoned. They knew that God was on their side and they were comforted by the prayers of the brethren.

Severely depressed people, on the other hand, are often guilty of generalizing and exaggerating their oppression. If a few people ignore them or treat them in a hostile way, then (in their minds) *everyone* is ignoring them and mistreating them. They often feel as if everyone is out to get them and nobody cares about them. This frequently causes a feeling of intense loneliness and alienation from others; they feel forsaken.

Finally, Paul wrote that they were "*struck down*, but not destroyed." In other words, there were occasions in their ministry when they were knocked off their feet by their difficulties. They most likely experienced setbacks and unforeseen events that caught them off guard and caused them to wonder how they were going to proceed. They felt their spiritual legs buckling underneath them at times, but they never allowed themselves to be destroyed by these things.

The severely depressed person not only perceives that they have been struck down, but they see themselves as being down *and out*. They think their life is in such disarray that there is little hope of it ever being put back together again. Because they are so firmly convinced of this grim and hopeless outcome, they simply quit. They are not merely struck down; they are knocked out.

John Bunyan's Description of Depression

John Bunyan described the experience of depression very accurately and vividly in his well-known allegory, *The Pilgrim's Progress.* At a certain point in their journey, Christian and his companion, Hopeful, found themselves on the property of Giant Despair:

> The giant got up early the next morning, and walking up and down his grounds, he spotted Christian and Hopeful sleeping there. Then with a fierce, threatening voice he woke them up and demanded where they had come from and what they were doing on his property. Christian and Hopeful answered shakily that they were pilgrims and that they had lost their way. The giant said, "You have committed an offense against me by trampling in and lying on my property last night. Therefore, you must come with me."[6]

Bunyan shows us here that Christian and Hopeful were captured and controlled by depression. In their minds, they had no choice but to submit because the Giant Despair seemed to have them by the throat. Knowing they were guilty of a wrong (trespassing), they were overpowered by their emotions and had little to say in their own defense:

> The Giant forced them to walk in front of him until they reached the castle. There he threw them into a very dark dungeon without any light which the two men found disgustingly foul and smelly. They lay there from Wednesday morning until Saturday night without even a crumb of bread. Christian felt doubly sorrowful because it was his ill-advised haste that had brought them into this distress.

Here we see the characteristic lack of appetite and inability to see beyond the moment of people who are experiencing depression. Everything around them seems dark and hopeless.

Bunyan went on to describe how the giant would come down to the dungeon and, without the slightest provocation, beat them unmercifully. Between beatings, the two men would lie helplessly on the floor, unable to move, with barely the strength to grieve their miserable condition. Finally, the giant went down to them with a knife, rope, and poison and advised them to kill themselves by saying, "You choose which means of death you prefer. Why should you choose life, seeing that it involves so much bitterness and pain?" Such is the experience of a person who is severely depressed.

A Contemporary Example

One severely depressed woman described her personal experience in this way:

> "Depression is your own private little hell, unknown to everyone but you and the Lord. It is very painful– the most devastating thing I've gone through. It makes one feel helpless and hopeless. The hurt at times is unbelievable, and apart from the grace of God, unbearable. It does not just go away with the passing of time. It is a real struggle, and lots of times you don't want to struggle anymore. Depression is very tiring,

and almost everything you do takes a tremendous amount of effort—even just getting out of bed some days.

"Depression robs you of your energy, your affections, your happiness, contentment, reasoning, etc. It leaves you bewildered, confused, sad, angry, sometimes resentful, sometimes tearful, anxious and nervous, with your "stomach in knots." It affects you physically; I lost 18 pounds, and I had a terrible skin rash for almost three years. It affects you mentally; you think of nothing except how badly you feel and what a waste your life is. It affects you spiritually; sometimes I've almost lost my assurance of salvation. I have felt forgotten and forsaken by God. It is difficult to pray, and when praying, it seems sometimes as if the prayer can't get past the ceiling.

"In depression, one sad thought leads to another, and in a very short period of time you are in the depths of despair. Crying is a commonplace experience for me. Even now as I write, I am crying and it's very difficult to break this habit. Crying doesn't relieve the hurt. In fact, it makes it worse and the result is more despair.

"Oh, God, I hurt so badly. I've heard of people dying of a broken heart, but this is worse. I'm living with a broken heart. I am so alone—please God, please let me die. My heart is heavy almost all the time and I forget what it feels like to be happy and content. I know we're not to ask "why," but I wish I had died 20 years ago when I had a serious medical problem. The last 20 years in between were not worth the last three years of suffering."

The Physical Effects of Depression

As we can see from the previous examples, severe depression has a marked effect on the physical body of those experiencing it. In an article on depression published in *The Journal of Pastoral Counseling*, Robert Smith, M.D., described severe depression and its effects on the body in this way:

"Depression is one of the conditions with much halo data. [*"Halo data" are the symptoms or manifestations of depression that can be physically observed.*] The first place to look is the most obvious–the counselee's face. His face literally oozes a "what's the use" attitude. His eyelids tend to droop; the corners of his mouth are turned down and seem to pull the entire facial expression down with them. His face is long, grim and sad. He appears listless and generally expresses an air of helplessness or hopelessness. Written on his face is what is going on inside him.

"All other visual and auditory clues or data follow the same pattern. His voice is quiet, and his speech tends to be slow. His voice is a monotone, and he uses little or no expression. As he talks, tears may come to his eyes. He may not look at the counselor; he may look at the floor instead. His hands press limply in his lap. He sits with a droop to his shoulders as though pushed down by the weight on his shoulders and the corners of his mouth. There's very little body motion as he talks. He walks slowly and at times almost shuffles. There's little "life spring" or bounce that shows some expenditure of energy. He is interested in doing what he does with as little effort as possible.

"This describes classic [*what we are calling "severe"*] depression. All these things are not always present, but there will be varying degrees of some of the signs present in most depressed people. Occasionally a [*severely*] depressed person displays the exact opposite signs. He is overactive, fidgety, and irritable, and he talks fast, but with disconnected speech. However, his physical symptoms are those of classic [*severe*] depression.

"The things that a [*severely*] depressed person complains of, and the physical changes that are present in his body, are identical to what is observed on the outside. He complains of having no pep or energy, and is always tired. He doesn't sleep well because he either has difficulty falling asleep or else he awakens early.

The latter is the most common complaint. Even when such a person does sleep, he awakens in the morning feeling as though he hasn't slept all night. Then he drags through the day fighting the fatigue and sleep, only to end up in bed that night, again unable to go to sleep. When he does, he typically spends it in restless sleep and awakens early and tired the next morning. He may have a sick headache in the morning, and sore feet and a little backache in the evening. He has no appetite and food does not look good to him. He only eats because he knows it's necessary. He may have lost some weight. In association with this, he complains of constipation. His mouth is dry and has a bad taste. He has lost interest in sex as well as other things that at one time were very important to him.

"The Lord made our bodies with automatic regulating systems controlling many of their functions. This system works something like the thermostat in our homes. When the temperature is low, the thermostat tells the furnace to put out more heat and the house warms up. When the temperature is high, the thermostat tells the furnace to quit putting out heat and so it stops. The thermostat for the autonomic (automatic) nervous system (ANS) is the brain and the spinal cord. Certain needs within the body tell the ANS to make certain changes. Such things as the activity of the intestinal tract, the amount of saliva produced by the mouth, sweating, the heart rate, and many, many others are controlled by the ANS. Even though all the functions are automatic, the brain can affect them. By "brain" is meant the reactions the human being has to the various experiences in his daily life. These reactions affect the ANS. This dynamic is what is going on in the depressed person. ...The intestinal tract slows down, producing loss of appetite, some nausea, indigestion, and constipation. Decreased food intake and decreased digestion produce weight loss. Decreased production by the salivary glands produces a dry mouth, which contributes to the bad taste. The entire metabolism slows down, producing lack of pep and energy, a condition encouraged by the lack of sleep.

"The tired, run down feeling may also be caused by the failure to rest while sleeping. When the depressed counselee goes to bed, he takes his problems with him. He thinks about them, tries to solve them and generally continues his daily activities in his mind. It is as though he is trying to sleep by a television set that is depicting his problems and activities. Even with the sound turned down or off, sleep is difficult and rest is impossible."[7]

PUTTING IT ALL TOGETHER

Any attempt to understand depression must be comprehensive in its view of the problem. As we have seen in the many examples given, depression includes and affects every aspect of a person's life; their physical body, emotions, behavior, intellect/cognition, theology, and history.

It is *physical*, in that it is often the cause of real physical difficulties such as extreme fatigue, insomnia, and loss of appetite. It is *emotional*, in that it is characterized by feelings of disappointment, sadness, discouragement, gloom, despondency, apathy, anxiety, anger, frustration, loneliness, emptiness, disillusionment, dejection, and despair. Depressed people are often controlled by their feelings and tend to practice "emotional reasoning;" that is, they consider their personal feelings to be accurate and valid above all else. Emotions become excuses for not fulfilling responsibilities or living in obedience to God's commands.

Depression is *behavioral*, in that it leads to inactivity, abdication of responsibility, and sinful actions and reactions. Depressed people commit sins of omission (not doing what they should do) and of commission (doing what they should not do). They sin with their mouth as well as their eyes, ears, hands, and feet. Frequently, depression affects how people interact socially, causing them to withdraw, place blame, misinterpret words and actions, and become excessively dependent on a few individuals. They are completely self-centered in their approach to most interpersonal relationships.

Depression is *intellectual*, or *cognitive*, in that people lose sight of God's purposes, goodness, wisdom, and power for salvation. They tend to think negatively of God, the world, the future, other people and themselves. The perceived enormity and hopelessness of their problems dominates all of their thinking. It is *theological*, in that it is associated with a distorted, deficient or defunct view of God and of their relationship with God.

Finally, depression is *historical*, in that it is often the result of a "snowball effect" in a person's life. In other words, a mild depression of the past–triggered by one or several events that actually happened or were perceived to have happened–was not handled properly and became a moderate depression. The moderate depression was not handled properly and became a severe depression. People who are not practiced in responding biblically to life's problems develop destructive life patterns that perpetuate, enlarge and intensify small problems to such a degree that they become very big and very serious ones.

In resolving any problem in life, including depression, the first step involves accurately defining the problem. An inaccurate or inadequate diagnosis of a problem usually leads to an inaccurate or inadequate solution. In this chapter, we have discussed and explored the nature of severe depression. These insights and ideas are meant to help us correctly identify and understand this kind of depression. If you (or someone you know and want to help) are struggling with depression, take some time to honestly and thoughtfully answer the following questions:

1. What are the *physical manifestations* of this depression?

   Review the examples in this and the last chapter (Asaph, Jeremiah, David, Ezekiel, etc.). Reflect on the statements regarding the way in which these people were affected physically by their depression, and identify any similarities to what is happening in your life or in the life of the person you want to help.

2. What are the *emotional components* of this depression?

   What words would accurately describe the feelings being experienced–disappointed, sad, discouraged, gloomy, miserable, despondent, anxious, angry, frustrated, apathetic, lonely, empty, disillusioned, dejected or despairing? Does the person tend to be constantly taking their emotional temperature? Do they practice "emotional reasoning," which is viewing their emotions as being trustworthy, dependable, and accurate reflections of reality?

3. What *behaviors or actions* seem to be connected to the depression?

    What actions have been taken or not taken as a result of the depression? What behaviors have increased or decreased with the depression? What impact or effect has the depression had on the person's relationships with people, the fulfillment of responsibilities, etc.?

4. What are the *intellectual* or *cognitive* aspects of this depression?

    What repetitive thoughts, perspectives, interpretations or mindsets are involved?

5. What *theological* impact has this depression had on this person's life?

    How has their attitude toward spiritual things been affected by their depression? How has their depression impacted their spiritual life? How do they view God?

6. What are the *historical* factors of this depression?

    Has it occurred previously? What was going on when it began? How long has it lasted? Has it gotten better or worse? In what circumstances, places or times does it improve or get worse? What effect have unpleasant circumstances or events had on the person? What are the typical ways in which they have handled and responded to their feelings in the past? Has there been a progression in the intensity and depth of their responses to distasteful occurrences?

    Determining the answers to these six sets of questions is a good starting point for overcoming the problem of depression, but it is only the *beginning*. In the next chapter, we will study a biblical perspective on the various factors that may facilitate the development of depression. Before moving on to the next chapter, however, I encourage you to spend some time thinking about and answering the following questions:

QUESTIONS FOR DISCUSSION AND APPLICATION:

1. What biblical examples were given of the third category of depression?

2. What are some of the symptoms of this kind of depression?

3. What is meant by the statement that the third category of depression is one of the conditions with much halo data?

4. Describe the difference between Paul's experience in 2 Corinthians 4:6-9 and the third category of depression.

5. What is the main point of the section in this chapter entitled, "Putting it All Together"?

6. What did you learn about depression from reading and studying these first two chapters?

7. Which of the Bible passages or examples used in this chapter was most interesting and meaningful to you in understanding depression? Why was this passage or example most meaningful?

8. Have you ever encountered someone experiencing one of the three kinds of depression described in this chapter? Which category of depression was this person experiencing? Describe how depression affected this person–physically, emotionally, behaviorally, intellectually/cognitively, spiritually, and historically.

9. Have you ever personally experienced any of the three types of depression? Which category of depression have you experienced? Describe how you were affected by your depression–physically, emotionally, behaviorally, intellectually/cognitively, spiritually, and historically.

10. What can you personally, or for the sake of helping others, learn about overcoming depression from the Bible passages and examples used in these chapters?

11. Do you agree with the statement that some discouragement and disappointment is to be expected in this sinful world? Why do you agree or disagree?

12. How prone are you to constantly taking your emotional temperature and allowing your feelings to control your life? When have you done this? When have you deliberately not done this?

13. Why is being ruled or controlled by your feelings a dangerous practice?

Chapter 3
Why Do People Get Depressed?

An understanding of how depression affects a person's life is very helpful in overcoming the problem of depression–whether mild, moderate or severe. In the last chapter, we discussed the fact that severe depression touches nearly every aspect of a person's life; their physical body, emotions, behavior, intellect, theology, and history. This is a crucial part of addressing the problem because the impact of depression on each of these areas must be understood and addressed. Though we often think of depression as a highly emotional experience, it is a mistake–indeed, a hindrance–to merely focus on the depressed person's emotions.

In addition to understanding these six aspects of a person's life and how they are impacted by depression, it is important to determine the various causes or occasions for depression. Knowing the cause of the problem is necessary for developing an appropriate biblical strategy for its solution. Since the Bible indicates that depression can be brought on by any of several different things, the solution must be tailored to fit their needs.

In this chapter, we will start by looking at a general biblical perspective on the fundamental cause of depression. Later, we will explore in depth three of its more specific causes. While all three of these causes may not be at work in every person's depression, at least one will be. In chapters four and five, we will study what God's solution to this problem is and how our knowledge of the specifics involved in a particular person's depression can help in designing a personal plan for overcoming their problem.

A GENERAL BIBLICAL PERSPECTIVE ON
THE CAUSES OF DEPRESSION

Why has depression become such a commonplace experience for people in this world–both today and for ages past? What are the theological roots of depression? How did depression become a part of human experience in the first place? As we seek to answer these questions biblically, the following truths seem to emerge as foundational to a correct analysis of the problem of depression:

First, *the experience of any kind of depression (mild, moderate or severe) is only possible in a fallen world.* Prior to the fall and the entrance of sin into creation and the hearts of men, there was nothing in our created world or in us that would have caused depression. "God saw all that He had made, and behold, *it was very good*" (Genesis 1:31). [Genesis 3:1-31; Romans 5:12-21; Romans 8:18-24.]

Second, *depression is the only logical, rationally consistent result of living without God.* If a person believes that the God of the Bible exists, but does not acknowledge Him as Savior and Lord, that person has a good reason to be depressed. If a person believes that God exists, but has a deficient understanding of how sinners are justified, or a deficient understanding of who and what God is, he also has every reason to be depressed.

The person who does not believe that God exists has every reason to be depressed because he has no absolute standard for determining anything in his life; values are relative and events are random. There is not, nor can there be, any purpose for his life, and sooner or later he discovers that. As a result, a logical and consistently thinking unbeliever cannot help but be depressed. "Remember that formerly you...were at that time separate from Christ...*having no hope and without God in the world*" (Ephesians 2:11-12). [Isaiah 8:19-20; Romans 1:18-32; Romans 15:4,13; Titus 1:2;]

Third, *deliverance from depression—which is one of the possible effects of the fall into sin—is made possible through the redeeming work (justification and sanctification) of Jesus Christ and the regeneration (new birth and continual work) of the Holy Spirit in us.* At salvation, we become new creatures in Christ. We are forgiven of our sins, restored to a right relationship with God, and transferred out of Satan's kingdom and into the kingdom of Christ Jesus. We are released from the bondage of sin, given the liberty of God's children, and given a new and proper perspective on ourselves, the world, and our future.

The renewal of the Spirit gives us new desires, comfort, security, purpose, power for living, and hope for the future. Because we have died to the reigning power of sin in our lives and been raised again to walk in newness of life, we enjoy all kinds of spiritual blessings in the heavenly places in Christ Jesus. And we have the assurance that God is working all things together for our good. [Romans 6:1-23; Romans

8:1-16, 26-39; 1 Corinthians 6:9-11; 2 Corinthians 5:17; Ephesians 3:1-23; Titus 3:3-7.]

Fourth, *experiential deliverance from depression (and other effects of sin) is not an automatic result of the regeneration and redemption that begins at salvation.* A true believer has the potential to experience deliverance from moderate and severe depression, but this deliverance is not spontaneously or effortlessly experienced and maintained.

Redemption and regeneration make it possible to be delivered from the temptations and struggles of sin. Through salvation, the believer is given all the resources needed for overcoming sin and the assurance of God's power to use those resources. However, the believer must still exercise his will in faithfully applying those resources to his benefit. [2 Corinthians 4:1-18; Ephesians 4:22-24; Philippians 2:3-8, 12-13; Philippians 4:8; Hebrews 12:1-4; James 1:2-5.]

Fifth, *because we all still struggle with indwelling sin, it is possible for believers to experience all three kinds of depression.* None of us have perfectly or continuously put off our old nature, which is corrupted by sin, and put on our new nature, which is created in true righteousness and holiness. Until we are fully transformed into the image of Christ, we will continue to struggle with old sin patterns, thoughts, values, and desires.

As long as we live in this sinful world, we will be tempted by difficult circumstances and sinful people and we will be affected by the work of Satan and his demons. All of these things make depression a very real *possibility* for those of us who know Christ as Savior and Lord. [Romans 6:10-19; Galatians 5:16-21; Ephesians 2:1-3; Ephesians 6:10-18; Colossians 3:1-17; James 1:13-16; 1 Peter 2:1, 11-12; 1 Peter 5:8.]

Sixth, *believers can look forward to a time when they will experience complete and continuous deliverance from all sin and all problems, including all kinds of depression.* In Heaven, there will be no depression of any kind or even the possibility of depression. All of the factors that create depression on earth will be totally removed in Heaven. The book of Revelation describes Heaven in this way:

> For this reason, they are before the throne of God; and they serve Him day and night in His temple; and He who sits on the throne will spread His tabernacle over them. They will hunger no longer, nor thirst

anymore; nor will the sun beat down on them, nor any heat; for the Lamb in the center of the throne will be their shepherd, and will guide them to springs of the water of life; *and God will wipe every tear from their eyes* (Revelation 7:15-17).

And He will wipe away every tear from their eyes; and there will no longer be any death; there will no longer be any mourning, or crying, or pain; the first things have passed away. And He who sits on the throne said, "Behold, *I am making all things new*" (21:4-5).

There will no longer be any curse; and the throne of God and of the Lamb will be in it, and His bond-servants will serve Him; they will see His face, and His name will be on their foreheads. And there will no longer be any night; and they will not have need of the light of a lamp nor the light of the sun, because the Lord God will illumine them; and they will reign forever and ever (Revelation 22:3-5).

In his book, *The Glory of Heaven*, John MacArthur explained that one day, for the believer in Christ, there will be no need for police or military forces because there will be no criminals, murderers, or thieves. There will be no wicked, violent, abusive, or selfish people. The curse that came as the result of sin "will be overturned and erased forever, with all its painful and detestable ramifications. Pain, the agony of toil, sweat, thorns, disease, sorrow, and sin will have no place whatsoever in Heaven."

At that time, the environment in which we live will be the best it could be. There will be no more thorns or thistles, earthquakes, hurricanes, droughts, or floods. All of these frightening and stressful things will be gone forever. No defect of any kind (spiritual, physical, emotional, mental, relational, motivational) will be found in any believer. In Heaven we will experience perfect pleasure, perfect knowledge, perfect comfort, perfect love, perfect joy, perfect relationships and perfect fellowship with God.[8]

In other words, we Christians can look forward to a time when all of the things that cause depression will be gone forever. That is the glorious promise of God to His children. Meanwhile, because of the effects of sin, depression remains a possible experience for believers as well as unbelievers. [For more on Heaven, see: Isaiah 65:17-19;

1 Corinthians 15:51-53; Philippians 3:20-21; 2 Peter 3:13; 1 John 3:2; Revelation 20:10; Revelation 21:8, 27.]

THREE SPECIFIC CAUSES OF DEPRESSION

A careful study of various biblical examples of depression indicates that depression can result from one of three specific causes (or some combination of these three). These three causes for depression are refusing to deal with sin and guilt, mishandling a difficult event, and having unbiblical standards or values. We will study each cause carefully.

1. Refusing to Deal with Sin and Guilt

Depression may be the result of unresolved sin and guilt in the life of an individual. Often the road to this kind of depression looks something like this:

1. *A sin is committed.* There are two basic ways we sin: we disobey God in some way by not doing what He commands, or we disobey God by doing what He forbids.

2. *We feel accused by either our conscience or other people.* When we have done something wrong, our conscience begins to accuse us of the wrong that we have done (Romans 2:14-15). Alternately, or in addition to that, someone in our life may point out our sin to us.

3. *We experience guilt and internal distress over our mistake.* Because of the accusation of our conscience or other people, we judge ourselves to be guilty and experience distress over that guilt.

4. *We delay confession and repentance of our sin.* It may also happen that these feelings of guilt and distress cause us to delay dealing with our sin. By failing to deal with the sin right away, guilt increases as we think about what we did wrong, the fact that we have been accused of that wrong, and the fact that we have not done anything about it.

5. *The growing guilt and distress caused by our conscience leads to depression.* Continuing to think about our sin and ignoring the appeals of our conscience (Romans 2:14, 15) to deal properly with it, we become depressed.

The two diagrams that follow depict how this kind of depression develops:

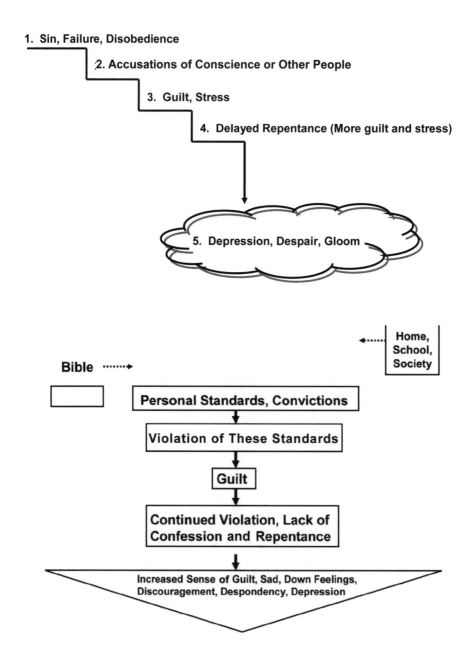

1. Sin, Failure, Disobedience

2. Accusations of Conscience or Other People

3. Guilt, Stress

4. Delayed Repentance (More guilt and stress)

5. Depression, Despair, Gloom

Home, School, Society

Bible

Personal Standards, Convictions

Violation of These Standards

Guilt

Continued Violation, Lack of Confession and Repentance

Increased Sense of Guilt, Sad, Down Feelings, Discouragement, Despondency, Depression

This was Cain's primary cause for depression in Genesis 4. Cain disobeyed God by offering an unacceptable sacrifice. He brought to God an offering of food he had grown, but God had made it clear that a blood sacrifice was necessary. (Though this is not stated explicitly in Genesis 4, the rest of Scripture makes it clear that remission of sin comes only by the shedding of blood.) We do know for sure that Cain did not bring the *best* offering because the Bible says, "...for Cain *and for his offering* He had no regard. So Cain became very angry and *his countenance fell*" (4:5).

It is likely that Cain's own conscience was rebuking him for his sin, though this is not stated explicitly in Scripture. Adam and Eve, Cain's parents, were well acquainted with the dire consequences of ignoring God's commands and it seems likely that they would have taught their children what they learned themselves the hard way. After Adam and Eve's sin in the garden, God provided a covering of animal skins for them. This is the first example in Scripture of blood sacrifice for the forgiveness of sin. Most likely, Cain knew very well that God desired an offering of an animal sacrifice from him.

Whether or not his conscience rebuked him, God clearly did. As we read in verse seven, God said to Cain: "Why are you angry? And why has your countenance fallen? If you do well, will not your countenance be lifted up? And if you do not do well, sin is crouching at the door; and its desire is for you, but you must master it" (4:7). God told Cain that he needed to walk in obedience in order to overcome his depression and to restore his relationship. He also warned him what would happen if he failed to obey.

As we know, Cain chose not to obey, and his hardened heart led him into greater sin and greater depression. After killing his brother and being again condemned by God, he cried out, "My punishment is too great to bear! Behold, You have driven me this day from the face of the ground; and from Your face I will be hidden, and I will be a vagrant and a wanderer on the earth, and whoever finds me will kill me" (4:13-14). Cain's sin and his failure to deal with it caused him to despair of his life.

David took this road to depression as well. In the last chapter, we looked at Psalm 32 in which David described the depression he was experiencing. He wrote, "*When I kept silent about my sin,* my body wasted away through my groaning all day long" (32:3). Many Bible scholars believe that this was the sin of adultery that David refused to deal with for possibly as long as a year. After committing adultery with Bathsheba, he had her husband, Uriah, killed on the battlefield so that no one would find out about the sin that he had committed (2 Samuel 11).

During this time of guilt and cover-up, David experienced great anguish and depression because of the accusation of his conscience and because, for a time, he refused to confess and repent. His depression was tied directly to his sin and his failure to deal with it properly. Psalm 32 indicates that when he finally repented of his sin, he experienced forgiveness, freedom from guilt, and a renewed sense of the joy of the Lord (32:5-11).

This was also the experience of Judas, the disciple who betrayed Christ. In Matthew 27, the Bible says, "Then when Judas, who had betrayed Him, saw that He had been condemned, *he felt remorse...*" (27:3). Judas' conscience condemned him and caused him to feel guilty. But instead of confessing his sin and repenting, it is apparent from Scripture that Judas refused to deal properly with his sin. He became so distressed by his guilt that he took his own life (27:5). Once again, depression resulted from sin and failure to deal properly with that sin.

I counseled a depressed woman who came into my office with her husband. As I talked with her, I learned that at the age of twelve, she had been diagnosed by a secular psychologist as a "catatonic schizophrenic," and had attempted suicide a few times. By the time I met with her, she was twenty-five and had been struggling with depression for about thirteen years. At that point, her doctors had abandoned talk therapy and her only "treatment" was various anti-depressant drugs.

As the three of us talked together, I discovered that this woman had been very sexually promiscuous as a young girl and continued to be as a young, married woman. Her husband dismissed her actions as simply a result of her "sickness," saying that she was not responsible for what she had done. I eventually challenged him with the fact that the Bible called her actions sin, not sickness.

After I said that, I turned to the young woman and asked if *she* thought that she was responsible for what she had done. When she said "yes," I counseled her to deal with her sin as God commands–by calling it sin, confessing it, and asking for forgiveness. That day in my office, she asked for forgiveness, and that step was the beginning of real change in her life.

So often today, we are told that our wrong actions are the result of sickness, not sin. Doctors can deal with sickness, but they have nothing to offer for sin. Only Jesus can deal with sin. But while the forgiveness is immediate, healing from the effects of the sin takes time. That woman's mind and behavior were not instantly transformed that day she accepted Christ, but the process of renewal had begun. Over time, we worked together on her habits and patterns of thinking. Her depression slowly lifted as she became a new person in Christ.

I worked with another woman who had also been through secular psychology and had attempted suicide on three occasions. Her "treatment" had included electric shock therapy which led to a great deal of memory loss. A Christian physician she later met encouraged her to get some biblical counseling. When she came to me, I asked her some questions about her relationships with her husband, children, and parents.

As we investigated many different areas of her life, we discovered that she was not living biblically in any of them. I took her to the Word of God and showed her the connection that often occurs between our failures (sin) and our feelings (guilt). This was all new to her! When she recognized and acknowledged the hold her failures and feelings had on her, she realized that she felt depressed because she was living in sin and feeling guilty about it.

This truth applies to all believers, whether we are experiencing depression or not. We cannot feel good when we are being rightly accused of our sin. When we are not relating to our spouses, or children, or parents, or others in a godly way, we will experience some amount of distress and guilt in our lives. When we are not fulfilling our responsibilities as we should, we will experience distress and guilt. The only way to relieve that distress and guilt and to experience true joy is to ask for forgiveness daily, and to live in obedience to God's Word.

2. Mishandling a Difficult Event

Depression may be the result of mishandling a hard or unpleasant situation. All too often when problems arise or disappointments confront us, we allow ourselves to focus on the unpleasant things around us or within us. We begin to replay them over and over again in our mind until they become our automatic thoughts. Or, we listen to our "friends" who commiserate with us and tell us how terrible our situation is, giving us encouragement in our brooding and self-pity. We become practical atheists who think, feel, and act as if God did not exist or at best practical deists, who act as if God did not care. Though we claim to believe in God and His perfect love, wisdom, sovereignty, and goodness, we deny it by the way we respond to our difficulties.

A study of Scripture reveals several examples of depression that arose from unbiblical responses to a difficult circumstance. In Numbers 11, Moses experienced constant criticism from the Israelites. He responded to this difficult situation by becoming greatly distressed. Moses revealed his depression when he asked the Lord to relieve him of both his leadership duties and his life. "I alone am not able to carry all this people, because it is too burdensome for me. So if You are going to deal thus with me, please kill me at once..." (11:14-15).

Likewise, Elijah responded wrongly to a difficult situation and became depressed. In 1 Kings 18, Elijah saw the Lord send down fire from Heaven to consume a drenched sacrifice. All of Israel, 450 prophets of Baal, 400 prophets of Asherah, and King Ahab saw it as well. Elijah probably expected all the people to repent and turn to the Lord after this powerful and miraculous event. Instead, after King Ahab told his wife, Jezebel, everything that Elijah had done (including the killing of all the false prophets), she promptly sent this message to Elijah, "So may the gods do to me and even more, if I do not make your life as the life of one of them by tomorrow about this time" (1 Kings 19:2).

Certainly this was not the response Elijah was hoping for or expecting. He had to have been disappointed and disillusioned by this difficult turn of events. And so, Elijah ran into the wilderness to escape what he thought was certain death at the hand of Jezebel. He collapsed under a tree and asked God to take his life. Instead of trusting in God for direction, protection, and comfort, Elijah relied on his own understanding (see Proverbs 3:5-6). His incorrect interpretation of events led to an ungodly response, and that response led directly to depression.

The following diagrams depict for us how this kind of depression develops. Each diagram depicts the downward path to the kind of depression that is facilitated by responding to difficult situations in an unbiblical way:

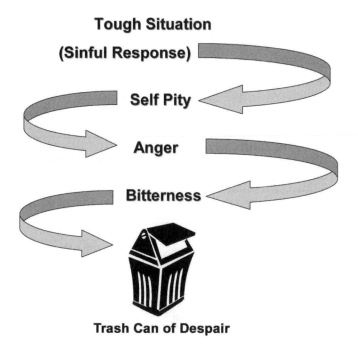

Tough Situation

(Sinful Response)

Self Pity

Anger

Bitterness

Trash Can of Despair

Diagram 2 gives us a picture of what goes on inside a person when he responds to difficult situations in an unbiblical way.

Depression can be serious, difficult, painful, and life-dominating

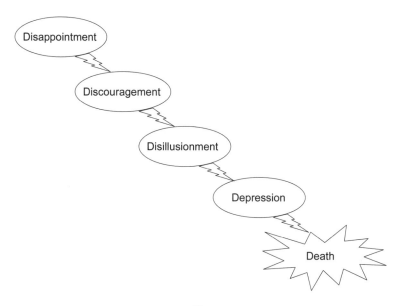

Disappointment

Discouragement

Disillusionment

Depression

Death

Diagram 3 illustrates the downward dynamic that occurs internally and behaviorally when people respond in an unbiblical manner to the pressures that come upon them from difficult circumstances:

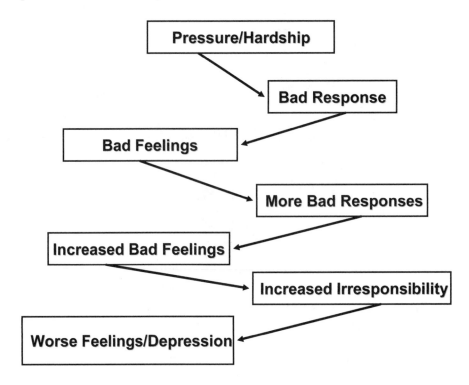

Difficulties that May Lead to Depression

There are many difficult circumstances that when handled incorrectly (unbiblically), can lead to depression. For example, the death of a loved one such as a spouse may be the triggering event for a person's depression. My wife's parents had been married fifty years when her father died. For fifty years, my mother-in-law had spent nearly every day with this man, sharing their lives in almost every way. Needless to say, his death was an incredibly hard situation for her. It would have been easy for her to slip into depression after losing someone so special to her.

A terminal illness can be the difficult event that triggers depression. It may be a person's own disease or that of someone they love, but it is devastating nonetheless. Sometimes mothers become depressed when their children first leave home for college, career, or marriage. Losing one's job can also be an unpleasant event that leads to depression.

A significant move can be an occasion for depression. I counseled an elderly couple that was forced to move (for financial reasons) out of a community they had lived in all their lives. They both were experiencing depression as a result of that move because it took them away from friends and neighbors they had grown to love and the house where they had raised their children. They struggled with depression for two years before coming to me for counseling.

A bad accident or a divorce is a difficult situation that can lead to depression. Sometimes, severe criticism from a loved one can trigger depression. Retirement can lead to depression because a person suddenly feels unproductive, unconnected, and unneeded. Young people can become depressed after failure in school, rejection in a relationship, or unrealized dreams of making it onto a team or other exclusive group.

I knew a young man, a college graduate, who spent much of his time sitting in a chair at home, doing nothing and staring into space. As a young person, he had always had social problems because of poor hearing. People often considered him aloof because he had difficulty participating in conversation. He was also a bit clumsy and had no athletic, musical, or artistic talent. As a result, he felt that people did not respect or like him.

His mother told me that one of the events that led to his depression was that he did not graduate from college with honors as he had expected to. Because of the many disappointments and difficulties that he had experienced in his youth, he had hoped to find success and admiration in his college academic accomplishments. Though he did well in college, his failure to achieve the highest honors was a contributing factor to his depression as a young adult.

Sometimes, feeling overwhelmed by tasks and responsibilities is a difficult situation that leads to depression. In Deuteronomy 1:28-29, Scripture describes what happened to the Israelites before they entered the land of Canaan. Spies were sent out to size up the task before them. Most of the spies came back and reported to the Israelites that there were giants in the land. When the people heard the spies' report, they became discouraged because they were convinced that God was asking too much of them. "…Our brethren have made our hearts melt, saying, 'The people are bigger and taller than we; the cities are large and fortified to Heaven...'" (1:28).

In chapter one I briefly mentioned a time in 1968 when I personally went through a time of serious depression. At that time, I experienced many of the symptoms previously mentioned under the moderate category and some of the ones under the severe depression category. It happened when I encountered some very unpleasant events in my ministry. For many years I had devoted my life to preparing for full-time ministry and then actually engaging in it. Initially, things went well in the church I pastored, but then I began to experience a great deal of opposition and criticism that I thought was completely undeserved. Factions began to form in the church I was pastoring with pro Mack and against Mack groups beginning to form.

Every Sunday as I preached I would look out on a group of people who obviously were opposed to my ministry. After the sermon, I would often be met at the door by people who would nit-pick over something I did or didn't do during the week, or something with which they disagreed in the sermon. As this went on and continued, I became concerned about what was going to happen to the church. What was going to happen to my family? What should I do? Should I stay or leave? If I leave, how and where would I minister? How would I support my family? What would happen to the people who had responded positively to my ministry and were in agreement with my doctrinal convictions and philosophy of ministry? For me, this was one of the most difficult times in my life. I walked around with a very heavy heart. I could and did cry, very easily. I worried. I became easily annoyed. I lost my zeal and enthusiasm for the work I was doing. I was utterly devoted to ministry and it seemed to me as a young pastor that the future in ministry looked pretty bleak.

What was going on? I was mishandling a difficult situation. I was not letting God's Word richly dwell within me (Colossians 3:16). I was not believing the many promises, passages and examples of God's Word that apply to situations like this. I could have quoted Romans 8:28, 29 and 1 Corinthians 10:13 and James 1:2-5 and Job 23:10 and 2 Corinthians 9:8 and Psalm 55:22 and a host of other Scriptures that speak to situations like the one I was facing. However, quoting the verses and really believing them is not necessarily the same thing. The lens through which I was viewing my circumstances was "my own understanding" rather than the Word of God. I was not casting down my imaginations and every high thought that was opposed to the knowledge of God. I was not taking every thought captive and making it obedient to Christ (2 Corinthians 10:4, 5). The result of my mishandling this distressing and unpleasant situation was an extended period of depression.

That was 1968 and as I write this book it is almost forty years later. To the praise of God, I can honestly say He delivered me from that depression. And though I have faced many tough situations since then, I have never descended as deeply into the dark valley of depression as I did at that time. What helped me to overcome and avoid that kind of depression ever since? Well, that's what I'll be writing about in chapters five and six. I know what is written in those chapters is effective because it is based on Scripture given to us by a God who can't lie, and because following the directives in those chapters has brought many people out of depression.

Separating Occasion From Cause

We have described a few of many possible examples of difficult events or situations in people's lives that can put them in a position to be tempted by depression. Now it is important to note that none of these things can be said to have *caused* someone's depression. These are all occasions for, *but not causes of*, depression. Depression is caused by a person's *response* to an event in their life, not the event itself.

Often, depression starts when the person begins to feel trapped and helpless in their unpleasant situation or circumstance. For example, some women want to work on and improve their marriage, but their husband will not cooperate or make any effort. Some couples want their children to become Christians, but after years of praying and teaching, they see no evidence of spiritual fruit in the lives of their children. There are men who want to get a better paying job so that they can more adequately support their family, but their efforts to advance at work or find something else with better pay go nowhere. They feel locked into their present job and begin to worry about the future. All these feelings of helplessness can turn into depression.

There are many people in this world who have experienced similar events who have *not* become depressed. For example, my mother-in-law, though she deeply loved her husband, did not become depressed after his death. Since an event such as the death of a loved one can impact the lives of people differently, it must be the *person's reaction to the event*–not the event itself–that causes depression.

We might diagram a person's response to a difficult event in this way:

EVENT + INTERPRETATION = RESPONSE

When a person goes through a difficult situation in life and interprets it from a *biblical* perspective, they respond to it in a *biblical* way. That biblical response leads to spiritual growth and life. On the other hand, when a person goes through a difficult situation and interprets it from an *unbiblical* perspective–using their own or the world's wisdom, they respond to it in an *unbiblical* way. That unbiblical response can result in any number of problems, including depression.

It is critical to recognize the fact that how a person interprets and responds to an event in their life is the deciding factor in what happens next. If asked, many women who have lost their husbands and become depressed would say their depression was the result of their husband's death, but this is not really correct. In reality, they are depressed because of the unbiblical way in which they interpreted and responded to that event.

I once counseled a woman who was experiencing depression after her husband of many years died. As we talked, I learned what interpretations and reactions to this event were at the root of her depression. She was depressed, in part, because she was feeling guilty about having been a poor wife. She admitted to me that she had yelled at her husband, not cooperated with him, and not encouraged him spiritually. Because she was powerless to change any of that after his death, she felt very guilty and that guilt caused her depression.

Psalm 37:8 says, "...do not fret; it leads only to evildoing." When you fret about something, it means that you run it over and over in your mind, focusing on all the negative aspects of the situation. If a woman who has lost her husband chooses to brood over that event, thinking about how lonely she is and wondering how she will manage without him, she will only increase her discouragement.

As a result, she will probably find it harder to fulfill her daily responsibilities. The added guilt of this makes the situation worse. She finds herself being pulled into a downward spiral of fretting and guilt that drains her of energy. Often, new worries arise as her mind continues to focus on negative things. She discovers new aches and pains and wonders if she is getting sick. Because of her preoccupation with her troubles, she loses interest in interacting with friends and neighbors.

Eventually, feelings of hopelessness and uselessness dominate her life. She is depressed–not because her husband died, but because she *responded improperly* to her husband's death. The death of a loved one is an unquestionably difficult event in any person's life, but God has a plan for handling hard situations that leads to righteousness, not sin. The woman I just described followed her own path and reaped the results. "There is a way which seems right to a man, but its end is the way of death" (Proverbs 14:12).

While grief over a loved one's death is perfectly legitimate (1 Thessalonians 4:13), that sorrow should never bring believers to the point where they begin to think that life no longer has meaning and that God and His Word are not sufficient. My parents had a very good, committed marriage, but when my father died, my mother became a much stronger woman than she had been before because she learned to do things she had always relied on him to do.

After his death, my mother devoted herself to good works (1 Timothy 5:10) and found opportunities to minister in ways she had not been able to before. At the age of sixty-five, she became more active in the church because she finally learned to drive a car. When someone in the church was having a hard time because of a family death or illness, she moved in with them and took over chores and responsibilities that were difficult for them. She also continued to welcome visitors into her home and remained active in the church nursery.

My parents loved each other deeply, and my mother was very sorry when he died, but by the grace of God she interpreted his death as a part of God's plan for her life. Because she interpreted this difficult event in a biblical way, she was able to respond to it by continuing to live a fruitful life for the Lord. As a result, she was not tempted to become depressed. She believed and lived Romans 8:28-29 with all her heart.

We must always remember that depression is not an inevitable and unavoidable result of difficult circumstances or events. How we *react* to difficult circumstances can be a major factor in the development of depression. Understanding our own or someone else's depression requires an honest look at how circumstances have been handled in the past and are being handled in the present.

3. Having Unbiblical Standards

Third, *depression may be the result of having unbiblical standards or an unbiblical value system.* The world preaches its values to us all the time. We see it on television, hear it on the radio, and read about it in books and magazines. For example, the world holds in high esteem anyone it considers to be very intelligent and those with many academic degrees. From newspapers to car bumpers, we are reminded of who is on the A-list and who is on the dean's list.

Education certainly has a legitimate place in this world. Without a good education, it is difficult or impossible to get a job in many fields. Our emphasis on achievements in the academics shows the high value that we place on intelligence and learning. But the other side of this standard–the unspoken message to the rest of society–is this: "If you don't make the grade, you aren't worth as much." This may be the world's value system, but it should not be the Christian's value system.

Another thing that our world places great value on is beauty and youth. Television shows and commercials make this standard quite obvious with a constant bombardment of beautiful, young people with perfect hair, clothes, and bodies. Commercials are designed to make us feel inadequate and unattractive if we fail to buy and use the latest beauty product. It is almost unacceptable anymore to show the gray hair and wrinkles that are the inevitable results of aging.

When we lived in the south some years back, my wife and I went out for dinner one night and happened on a Miss Louisiana Pageant. The dressed-up and made-up ladies we saw that evening were not vying for a place in the Miss America Pageant, however, because they were only eight years old. Sadly, pageants such as these tell our young children that beauty and youth are of significant worth. Of course, the other side of this is that ugliness and commonness are not acceptable. There are no beauty contests for older women, or young girls with freckles, big noses, large bodies or other "imperfections". Females who accept these values may judge themselves to be inferior people and then begin to experience discouragement and depression.

Talent is also highly esteemed in our world today. Great musicians, star athletes, and popular entertainers are praised, adored, and showered with money and attention. Young children look up to these people as their "heroes" and dream of the day when they will put on the same uniform and get all the same attention.

Of course, not every young boy is going to make it to the Major Leagues. So what does the uncoordinated little guy in right field think about himself when his coach constantly praises the talented kid in left field who helped win the game, and barely acknowledges–or even yells at–him? If he thinks, as the world does, that his worth is tied to his athletic ability, he might very well struggle with depression at some point in his life.

Sadder than the world having these values is the fact that very often believers do as well. As a father, these wrong values affected me. My son played basketball, and when I was unable to see a game, I would ask him about it when he came home. "Nathan, how many points did you score? And how many points did Joe score?" I asked because I wanted to know if my son outscored Joe. With these questions, I communicated to my son that what mattered was how good a basketball player he was, and that was very wrong.

Do any of these things matter to Christ? Many Christians today share the world's values. They evaluate their worth on the basis of how they measure up to the world around them. If they find themselves deficient in any area–not intelligent, beautiful, young, or talented enough, they either expend great energy trying to change, or they simply give up and become depressed by their inadequacy. Both responses are wrong; the first one often leads to the second one (depression) because chasing perfection is a never-ending and highly unfulfilling task.

When our value system is worldly, we may be tempted to be envious or jealous of others who have more than we do because we think we deserve the same. Asaph's struggle with despondency, described in Psalm 73, was connected with self-pity arising from envy and jealousy. He wrote in that Psalm that there was a time in his life when "my feet came close to stumbling, my steps had almost slipped" (73:2). He was weary and thoroughly dejected.

How did he get to that point? Searching the passage, we find that he had become envious of others around him. Others were prospering and did not seem to have problems in their lives. What is more, they were prospering despite the fact that they were wicked, immoral, and ungodly people. As Asaph pondered these things, he started to feel sorry for himself. Out of his self-pity and envy came a spirit of depression.

Many people today are depressed for the same reason. Some time ago I received a call from someone who asked me if I would visit a woman who had been committed to the psychiatric ward of a local hospital. He told me she had tried to commit suicide on two previous occasions. In this latest instance, she had taken an overdose of pills.

During the course of my visits with her, I discovered that this woman was full of self-pity because she was now over forty years old and the Lord had not yet given her a husband. She desperately wanted to have a family. To make matters worse, her sister was married and had children. She envied her sister, and her envy had turned into bitterness and hatred toward her sister and, to some degree, God as well. She was depressed because of self-pity that originated with envy.

Many other unmarried women battle depression because they see other women getting married and having children. They desperately want to be wives and mothers, but for some reason God has not been pleased to give them a husband. Some time ago, a young woman heard me preach and came out of the church in tears. I had preached that morning on the subject of submitting to God's will.

She said to me, "God has really dealt with my heart. I very much want a husband and a family. Recently I have become somewhat bitter against God for not giving me that and I see now that I've been wrong. This morning I decided to tell God that I'm willing to accept and rejoice in whatever His will is for me. From now on, I'll leave the future to God and not let myself become consumed with desire for things He hasn't given me." Since then, though she still has occasional battles, she has become a much happier and useful person.

1 John 2:16 says, "For all that is in the world, the lust of the flesh and the lust of the eyes and the boastful pride of life, is not from the Father, but is from the world." When someone is motivated by the lust of the flesh, it means they seek happiness and fulfillment from physical pleasure, comfort and security. When someone is motivated by the lust of the eyes, it means they seek happiness and fulfillment from having material goods or from good looks or possessions or impressing people. And when someone is motivated by the pride

of life, it means they seek happiness and fulfillment from power, prestige, control, success, popularity and approval. If they are unable to get these things, or if anyone stands in their way of satisfying these desires, they can become angry, anxious, or depressed.

Our values are what we believe is important, what makes life worthwhile, and what we believe can really bring happiness and fulfillment to our lives. Diagram 1 depicts how these values impact us emotionally and can be a facilitator of depression:

DEPRESSION FLOWCHART

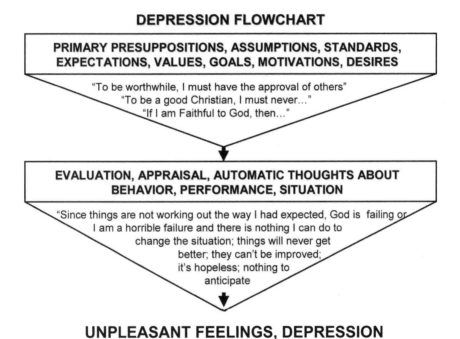

Diagram 2 illustrates what happens when we reject a biblical perspective on what is important and exchange what is really valuable and worthwhile, according to God, with what is a worldly and demonic perspective on values. The chart itself is an exposition of Romans 1:21-32 in diagram form which depicts what happens emotionally and behaviorally when men turn from their God-given purpose for living (glorifying God and enjoying Him forever) to living and valuing created things and values.

Having unbiblical standards can easily lead to unrealized or unrealistic expectations. Luke 24 tells us about two men who were very sad in heart. A spirit of heaviness had enveloped them. When Jesus approached and began to walk with them, the men were prevented somehow from recognizing Him. As they began to talk with Christ, they explained to Him that they were sad because they were hoping that Jesus Christ would redeem Israel. In essence, they admitted that their depression was the result of their unrealized hopes. They had put their hope in Christ, and when He died, their hope died as well.

Romans 1:21-32 in Diagram

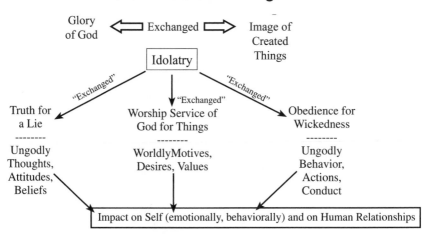

Sometimes, as believers, we may struggle to reconcile the conditions and problems of the world with what we know or think we know about God. This is another type of unbiblical thinking that can lead to depression. We look around us and say, "This world is such a mess!" But when we read the Scriptures, we are told that God is in control. Putting these two truths together–the rampant iniquity in the world and God's sovereignty–is difficult and confusing. As a result, we may come to God saying, "Lord, I know You are sovereign and in control, but why do You allow these things to go on? Why do You permit evil things to occur?" Our incomplete and sometimes wrong understanding of God and Scripture can result in depression. Several thousand years ago, the prophet Habakkuk struggled with this problem:

> How long, O Lord, will I call for help, and You will not hear? I cry out to You, "Violence!," yet You do not save. Why do You make me see iniquity, and cause me to look on wickedness? …Are You not from everlasting, O Lord, my God, my Holy One? We will not die. You, O Lord have appointed them to judge; and You, O Rock, have established them to correct (Habakkuk 1:1-2, 12).

What seems to be a paradox is still a problem for some of us in the twentieth century. Likewise, the writer of Psalm 77 seems to have been struggling with reconciling the evil around him with what He knew of God:

> Will the Lord reject forever?
> And will He never be favorable again?
> Has His lovingkindness ceased forever?
> Has His promise come to an end forever?
> Has God forgotten to be gracious,
> Or has He in anger withdrawn His compassion?
> Then I said, "It is my grief,
> That the right hand of the Most High has changed."
> (Psalm 77:7-10)

This psalmist had adopted an unbiblical way of thinking and had, as a result, become depressed.

The same could be said of Elijah's depression in 1 Kings 19. It is worth noting that this episode was an anomaly in Elijah's life. Elijah was a great man of God who trusted and obeyed his Lord most of the time. At this particular time, however, Elijah allowed himself to engage in some very unbiblical thinking and it caused a severe depression as we discussed in chapter two. Elijah's story is valuable in that it reminds us that what happened to him, one of the greatest prophets that lived, could just as easily happen to us.

As believers, we are called to "not be conformed to this world, but [to] be transformed by the renewing of [our] mind…" (Romans 12:2).

We have been given a different value system–God's system, and that system is very different from that of the world. This is why the apostle Paul could say in 2 Corinthians 12:10 that he was well content with weakness, insults, distresses and difficulties. Paul really believed that God works all things for good to those who love Him (Romans 8:28) and that God is faithful and will not allow us to be tempted beyond what we can bear (1 Corinthians 10:13).

In 2 Corinthians 4:8-11 we read that Paul was "afflicted in every way...perplexed....persecuted...struck down...constantly being delivered over to death." Why did he not succumb to depression in these awful circumstances? Paul told us in this same passage. He wrote that he knew he had been given a ministry and had received mercy (4:1). He also knew that his present sufferings were producing good–"an eternal weight of glory far beyond all comparison" (4:17). The apostle Paul avoided depression in the midst of terrible circumstances because he had a biblical, not worldly, value system.

I have counseled many people who were experiencing depression as a result of having unbiblical standards and values. When they compared themselves to what the world judges to be worthy, they found themselves severely lacking and therefore worthless. If John Bunyan had acted as they, we would very likely not have the great Christian allegory, *"The Pilgrim's Progress"* and other books he wrote in prison. Bunyan spent twelve and half years in prison while his family suffered in poverty because he refused to adopt the world's standards. Instead of becoming depressed or bitter, he studied the Scriptures intently and allowed God to use his difficulties for good. Adopting the world's way of thinking is an easy road to depression, but keeping our eyes fixed on Jesus is a sure way out.

A Combination of All Three

Sometimes, all three factors are at work to some extent in a person's depression. For example, someone might encounter a difficult circumstance and fail to respond to it in a biblical way. They forget that God works all things together for good (Romans 8:28-29), that God never allows His children to be tempted beyond what they are able to bear (1 Corinthians 10:13), and that trials are a way for believers to develop perseverance (James 1:2-4).

Because they are thinking unbiblically, a depressed person may then respond to their depression by doing or saying sinful things. In most cases where a person has committed an obvious sin, they did so because at the time they were thinking unbiblically, and it is likely they will fail to repent of that sin if they continue in their unbiblical thinking. Many of the scriptural examples used in previous chapters (Elijah, Moses, Cain, David) involve this combination of causes of depression.

For example, Cain sinned by not offering a pleasing sacrifice to the Lord. When God rebuked him for this, he became jealous and resentful of his brother, and bitter and angry against God. Instead of resolving his sin with God and responding biblically to the rebuke he had received, he made his situation far worse by killing his brother. Though unresolved sin was probably the primary cause, the other two factors were at work to some extent in Cain's depression as well.

It is important that we understand these major causes of depression because this is the key to overcoming the problem. So often depression is blamed on circumstances and other things outside of a person, but the truth is that these outer things are powerless to affect our hearts unless we allow them to. It is necessary for us to understand what truly underlies our own or someone else's depression (in most cases, unbiblical responses) so that these responses can be addressed. It is also important to determine what the original cause for depression was and what other causes are only complicating factors. The problem of depression will never be properly and completely solved unless the solution is directed at its true source.

A Word on Physical Causes

As I mentioned in the first chapter, there are a minority of cases in which depressed feelings are caused by a physiological problem. When seeking to determine the root causes of a person's depressed feelings, it is important to keep this possibility in mind. When a physical problem is, in fact, the cause, the person should be referred to a medical doctor for proper treatment. See Chapter 8, pages 142 and 143 for more on determining the likelihood of a physical cause for depression. But before you proceed to that chapter, I encourage you to spend some time thinking about and answering the following questions:

QUESTIONS FOR DISCUSSION AND APPLICATION:

1. What is a general biblical answer to the question of why people get depressed? What are the theological roots of depression?

2. Explain the statement that "depression is the only logical, consistent result of living without God". Why does the author say this is so?

3. What does the redeeming work of Christ have to do with deliverance from depression?

4. If the redeeming work of Christ is the ultimate solution to the problem of depression, why do believers still get depressed?

5. Explain why a refusal to deal with personal sin can be a cause of depression.

6. What biblical examples demonstrate the biblical accuracy of this statement?

7. Explain the statement that we become depressed because we function as practical atheists?

8. What biblical examples demonstrate the biblical accuracy of this statement?

9. Explain the statement that difficult circumstances may be the occasion of depression, but they are not the cause of depression.

10. Explain the meaning of the diagram,
EVENT & INTERPRETATION = RESPONSE.

11. What is meant by the statement that "depression may be the result of having unbiblical standards or values"?

12. What are some unbiblical values that people may have, and how does the adoption of these values connect to the problem of depression?

13. How do the truths expressed in 1 John 2:16 relate to the problem of depression?

14. Why is an understanding of the three specific causes of depression mentioned in this chapter an important aspect for preventing and overcoming depression?

15. Have you personally experienced a case of the blues in a moderate or severe way because of a failure to deal with your sin properly or because you responded to difficult circumstances in an unbiblical way or because you were being influenced by an unbiblical value system? Explain the specifics of the situations related to your moderate or severe case of the blues.

16. What have you personally, or for the sake of helping others, learned from this chapter about the causes of depression that will be helpful in your own life or in your ministry to others?

17. Do the things presented in this chapter as the causes of depression make biblical sense? In other words, are they supported by Scripture?

Chapter 4
Getting Out of the Blues-
Biblical Principles

A number of years ago our oldest son bought a large house in Philadelphia, Pennsylvania. The house had three floors and two staircases running between the floors. This meant, of course, that there was more than one way to go both upstairs and downstairs in the house. Though both staircases served the same basic function, they did so in somewhat different ways. One staircase was very steep, narrow, and had sharp turns while the other was very gradual, broad and had wide turns. Navigating these two staircases successfully required different approaches appropriate to their different construction.

There is a sense in which developing and defeating depression is like the staircases in that house. There is more than one way to go down into depression, as we noted in the last chapter. Some get to the basement of depression because of unresolved sin, some because they have mishandled a hard situation, and some because they are being influenced and controlled by unbiblical beliefs. The final destination is the same, though the path there may be different for different people.

Just as the path down can be different, the road out will be different as well. Once depression has been accurately diagnosed, it must be dealt with in a way appropriate to its cause. If someone is dealing with unresolved sin in their life, they will need different help to resolve their problem than someone who is mishandling a difficult situation.

Each person needs to confront the particular problem that led to their depression in order for that depression to be resolved. And those who counsel depressed people need to take heed that they do not become as Job's counselors–giving the right counsel to the wrong person–as Proverbs 18:13 warns against: "He who gives an answer before he hears, it is folly and shame to him."

Assuming that the problem has been accurately diagnosed, what approach is necessary for each of the three main causes of depression?

Since Christ is the source of "all the treasures of wisdom and knowledge" (Colossians 2:3), we must look to His Word for help. The Bible contains many important principles that equip us to deal with the various causes of depression.

THE UNIVERSAL REQUIREMENT

The unbeliever's ultimate problem in dealing with the problem of depression is that overcoming the kind of blues that are not directly related to some physical disease can only be accomplished with God's help. The Bible teaches us that man is utterly sinful. "As it is written, 'There is none righteous, not even one; there is none who understands, there is none who seeks for God" (Romans 3:10-11). "For all have sinned and fall short of the glory of God" (Romans 3:23). As a result of man's sinful nature: "...the hearts of the sons of men are full of evil and insanity is in their hearts throughout their lives" (Ecclesiastes 9:3). This sin has separated and alienated all people from God. "But your iniquities have made a separation between you and your God, and your sins have hidden His face from you so that He does not hear" (Isaiah 59:2).

The Bible's picture of our natural condition is black indeed, and it explains why we do not and cannot naturally obey God. By nature we are sinners; transgressors of God's law, and not rightly related to God. We are alienated from God, the true source of all joy and contentment. In this state, we are incapable of experiencing real joy and overcoming depression, and we never will until something happens to change that.

Changing our alienation from God is precisely what Jesus Christ came to do. God sent His only begotten Son into the world to deal with sin. Scripture says that Jesus Christ, as our representative, kept the law that we had not kept and could not keep. More than that, by His death on the cross, Jesus Christ paid the debt of every person who truly trusts in and submits to Him.

Jesus Christ came in the place of His people and satisfied every charge that God's law had against them. "God made Him who had no sin to be sin for us, so that in Him we might become the righteousness of God" (2 Corinthians 5:21). By His death on the cross, He paid our penalty and made it possible for us to come into a vital relationship with God. "But now in Christ Jesus you who were once far away have been brought near through the blood of Christ" (Ephesians 2:13).

God's way–the only way–of bringing sinners into a right relationship with Himself is through Jesus Christ. Jesus Christ is "the way, and the truth, and the life; no one comes to the Father but through" Him (John 14:6). So whenever we recognize our true condition (alienation from God), become truly sorry for our sinful life, and begin to depend on Jesus Christ, then God forgives us of our sin.

More than that, God puts the righteousness of Jesus Christ to our account and brings us into a very close relationship with Himself. "But as many as received Him, to them He gave the right to become the children of God, even to those who believe in His name" (John 1:12). "So then you are no longer foreigners and aliens, but you are fellow citizens with the saints, and are of God's household" (Ephesians 2:19).

In other words, reconciliation to God can only come through Jesus Christ, and that reconciliation is a vital and universal requirement for those who want to overcome depression. Apart from a restored relationship with God, we have every reason to be hopeless and depressed. Without Christ, we are cut off from God–our Creator, Sustainer, Sovereign and Judge. With Christ, we have a solid basis and reason for true and lasting hope and joy.

OVERCOMING DEPRESSION CAUSED BY UNRESOLVED SIN

The first specific cause of depression that we discussed was failing to deal in a biblical way with our sin. Using several of the psalms, the story of Cain's depression, and the story of Jonah's rebellion and later depression, I have gleaned the following list of steps for specifically dealing with this kind of depression:

1. If we are depressed because of our failure to deal with a particular sin, we must *specifically identify and acknowledge the sins and failures that are at the root of our struggle*. In Psalm 32 David described how his unconfessed sin caused him great physical anguish until he finally acknowledged it to God: "When I kept silent about my sin, my body wasted away through my groaning all day long...I acknowledged my sin to You, and my iniquity I did not hide" (32:3, 5a). As we do this, we need to carefully and honestly consider both sins of commission–things that we have done that we should not have–and sins of omission–things that we should have done

that we have not. 1 John 1:8 says, "If we say that we have no sin, we are deceiving ourselves and the truth is not in us."

2. We must *make sure we are using Scripture as our standard of right and wrong.* We cannot begin to think properly about our sin and our need for repentance unless we are basing our thinking on God's Word. We must understand that God's Word is the supreme authority in these matters (Isaiah 8:20) and that sin is lawlessness (1 John 3:4), and we must learn to hate sin as God hates sin. "Therefore I esteem right all Your precepts concerning everything, I hate every false way" (Psalm 119:128).

3. We must *be sure we understand the seriousness of our sin.* The prophet Nathan was sent to King David by the Lord because David did not understand the seriousness of his sin of adultery. Nathan told David a story that helped him to finally see how serious his sin really was (2 Samuel 12). Afterward David wrote, "Against You, You only, I have sinned and done what is evil in Your sight, so that You are justified when You speak and blameless when You judge" (Psalm 51:4).

4. We must *be sure that we understand what genuine repentance and confession requires.* Psalm 51 is a good picture of what true repentance looks like: demonstrating a true humility of spirit towards God (51:1), being willing to call sin the evil that it is in God's sight (51:2-3), having a true understanding of the seriousness of our sin and being willing to take personal responsibility for it (51:4), demonstrating a godly sorrow over our sin and a genuine desire for forgiveness (51:5-9), and desiring a changed heart—one that hates sin and loves godliness (51:10-12).

5. We must *understand the nature and basis of God's forgiveness—that it is freely given of grace through faith.* This understanding is important because it gives us hope for the future. There is nothing we can do to earn God's forgiveness, so there is no sin so great that it cannot be forgiven by our Heavenly Father. "In Him (Christ) we have redemption through His blood, the forgiveness of sins according to the riches of His grace" (Ephesians 1:7). Scripture indicates that once we have properly dealt with our sin through faith in Christ and His atoning work on the cross and through confession and repentance, we no longer need to be weighed down by guilt. God promises in Scripture to remember our sins no more (Jeremiah 31:34), to remove them as far as the east is from the west

(Psalm 103:12), and to cast them into the depths of the sea (Micah 7:19). God's forgiveness through Christ is free, all-sufficient, and everlasting.

6. We must *confess our sin to anyone who has been directly hurt by it and make restitution whenever possible.* That confession must, of course, start with God because our sin is always against Him first (Psalm 51:4). But our confession must also extend to the people who have been directly hurt by it: "Therefore, confess your sins to one another" (James 5:16a). More than that, if possible, we should make every effort to make restitution for our sin when it directly hurt or offended other people. This is what Zaccheus did when he met Jesus and became aware of his sin against many people: "'Behold, Lord, half of my possessions I will give to the poor, and if I have defrauded anyone of anything, I will give back four times as much'" (Luke 19:8).

7. We must *make a commitment to forsake our sin.* "He who conceals his transgressions will not prosper, but he who confesses and forsakes them will find compassion" (Proverbs 28:13). In other words, we must commit our mind and heart to putting off completely the sin we have been involved in and whatever thought patterns, attitudes, desires, and actions that went along with it. Christ's command to the adulterous woman is for us as well: "Go. From now on sin no more" (John 8:11).

8. We must *replace ungodly habits with godly ones.* It is not enough simply to stop doing evil; we must also commit ourselves to start doing good. The apostle Paul instructed the Ephesians in this when he wrote, "He who steals must steal no longer; but rather he must labor, performing with his own hands what is good, so that he will have something to share with one who has need. Let no unwholesome word proceed from your mouth, but only such a word as is good for edification according to the need of the moment, so that it will give grace to those who hear" (Ephesians 4:28-29). In each case Paul mentioned, sin was not just to be forsaken but also to be replaced by a specific act of obedience.

9. We must *demonstrate that we have learned from our failure by making plans to avoid and flee from any temptation to fall back into our sin.* Bad habits can be hard to break. If we are not prepared with a plan for how we will avoid temptation in the future, we may easily find ourselves entangled in old problems once again. It is difficult to

suddenly say "no" to something that we have been saying "yes" to for a while. It is vital, then, that we plan specific steps we will take to confront temptation so that we are able to overcome it.

As we make this plan, we must also *be sure that we understand God's provision for resisting temptation.* God has not left us to battle evil in our own strength; were that the case, we would surely fail. Rather, God shows us grace in that He promises to always provide a way of escape: "No temptation has overtaken you but such as is common to man; and God is faithful, who will not allow you to be tempted beyond what you are able, but with the temptation will provide the way of escape also, so that you will be able to endure it" (1 Corinthians 10:13). More than that, we are promised an abundance of grace to overcome: "And God is able to make all grace abound to you, so that always having all sufficiency in everything, you may have an abundance for every good deed" (2 Corinthians 9:8).

An important part of making a plan to overcome future temptation should also include *forming an accountability relationship with other believers.* After warning us to not let our hearts become callous toward sin, the writer of Hebrews said we should work to prevent this by being accountable to each other: "But encourage one another day after day, as long as it is still called 'Today' so that none of you will be hardened by the deceitfulness of sin" (3:13). Paul taught the same in Galatians: "Brethren, even if anyone is caught in any trespass, you who are spiritual, restore such a one in a spirit of gentleness...bear one another's burdens, and thereby fulfill the law of Christ" (6:1-2).

10. We must *take seriously Paul's admonition to forget what is behind and press forward to what God has for us ahead.* "Brethren, I do not regard myself as having laid hold of it yet; but one thing I do; forgetting what lies behind and reaching forward to what lies ahead, I press on toward the goal for the prize of the upward call of God in Christ Jesus" (Philippians 3:13-14). We have all failed in the past and we are all going to fail again, but once our sin has been properly dealt with before the Lord and with others, we must leave it behind and set our minds on what God wants from us today and each day after.

OVERCOMING DEPRESSION CAUSED BY MISHANDLING A DIFFICULT EVENT

Depression caused by a wrong response to difficult circumstances requires a different approach. The key to overcoming this depression is found in Philippians 4:4, where Paul wrote, "Rejoice in the Lord always; again I will say, rejoice!"

What did Paul mean by this command? Should we always have a smile on our face? Should we never mourn a loss? To understand what Paul meant by this command it will be helpful to note what Paul did *not mean* when he said to rejoice always. First, as we carefully consider these words, we should note that he did not say, "Rejoice, unless your life is in danger," or, "Rejoice, unless your responsibilities seem too great," or, "Rejoice, unless you have just lost a loved one," or, "Rejoice, unless your circumstances are very difficult." No, Paul said, "Rejoice...*always*...," which means in *all* circumstances, at *all* times, and in *all* places. Second, we know from the rest of Scripture that he did not mean that we ought to go around laughing and smiling all the time. I know some Christians who seem to think that we have to be constantly laughing or smiling. But that is not what Paul was talking about.

Certainly laughter is a good gift of God. Ecclesiastes 3:4 reminds us that there is "a time to weep and a time to laugh." In Psalm 126, the psalmist wrote, "When the Lord brought back the captive ones of Zion, we were like those who dream. Then our mouth was filled with laughter and our tongue with joyful shouting..." (126:1-2). That laughter was holy laughter and very pleasing in the sight of the Lord. In Proverbs 5:18-19, it says that husbands are to "rejoice in the wife" of their youth and to "be exhilarated always with her love." Fun and laughter ought to be a common occurrence in every Christian home, but that was not what Paul was talking about in Philippians 4:4.

Third, when Paul exhorted us to "rejoice always," he did not mean that we should never sorrow. He did not mean we should be happy when a loved one dies, or that we should laugh when we are criticized. Again, Ecclesiastes 3:4 teaches us that there is not only a time to laugh, but also a time to cry. In John 11, we learn that Jesus stood outside the tomb of Lazarus and wept. Christ also wept as He stood outside the city of Jerusalem and pronounced judgment on it (Luke 19:41-44). Whatever Paul meant by rejoicing always, he did not mean that we should never cry.

What then *did* Paul mean by this command? 1 Peter 1:3-6 sheds some light on this question. After describing some of the blessings believers have in Christ, Peter said, "In this you greatly rejoice, even though now for a little while, if necessary, you have been distressed by various trials" (1:6). This statement indicates that both rejoicing and sorrow can exist in the same heart at the same time. Paul said the same thing in 2 Corinthians 6:10 when he described the servants of God as being "...sorrowful yet always rejoicing." It is indeed possible to rejoice and to sorrow at the same time. Let us look briefly at two steps toward "rejoicing in the Lord":

Step 1: A Right Relationship

The key to understanding what Paul meant by the command "rejoice always," and how this provides the answer to the problem of depression caused by mishandling hard circumstances is found in the three words that follow "rejoice." Paul said that we are to "rejoice *in the Lord* always." This means we cannot rejoice in the Lord unless we are vitally related to Jesus Christ; unless we know Christ as our Savior and Lord. We cannot rejoice in someone with whom we have a bad relationship or no relationship at all.

Step 2: Obedience

Salvation through Jesus Christ is the basic requirement for overcoming any depression. But once we have a relationship with Christ, how do we go about changing our ungodly responses to difficult events so that we can overcome depression?

To answer this, we must look again at Philippians 4:4: "Rejoice in the Lord always; and again I say, rejoice." When Paul wrote these words as a command, he meant that rejoicing in the Lord was something that would require personal effort. In other words, it is not an automatic experience for believers. Though it is indeed *im*possible to experience true joy apart from the enabling of the Holy Spirit (Galatians 5:22), rejoicing in the Lord becomes our daily experience only by our own concerted effort and diligent practice. The indwelling Holy Spirit makes our efforts possible and successful, but the Spirit normally does not work apart from our efforts.

Consider the example of the man who was healed by Jesus in Mark 3:1-5. Jesus commanded this man to stretch out his hand before all the people in the synagogue. By God's power, this man was able to do what he could never have done on his own. But while his obedience was enabled by God, he still had to put forth the effort to obey.

In the same way, believers should never question their ability to obey God's commands because God has promised to give us the power to obey. "So then, my beloved, just as you have always obeyed...work out your salvation with fear and trembling; for it is God who is at work in you, both to will and to do for His good pleasure" (Philippians 2:12-13).

Since we know that the Holy Spirit has equipped us for every good work, we should hear God's commands and put forth the effort to immediately obey them. "...walk in a manner worthy of the Lord, to please Him in all respects, bearing fruit in every good work...strengthened with all power, according to His glorious might" (Colossians 1:10-11). This means that we must personally discipline ourselves to "rejoice in the Lord always," believing that regardless of our external circumstances or internal condition, the Holy Spirit will enable our obedience.

When we "rejoice in the Lord always," we daily choose to focus not on the problem and our feelings about it but on the solution and God's command to rejoice. We talk to ourselves instead of listening to ourselves; we walk by faith rather than sight; we focus on the unchangeable God and His Word rather than our changeable feelings. We think as David did in Psalm 16:8-9, "I have set the Lord continually before me; because He is at my right hand, I will not be shaken. Therefore my heart is glad and my glory [inner man] rejoices; my flesh also will dwell securely."

Of course, this is not to say that overcoming depression is as simple as cheering up because things could be worse, pretending our problems are not all that serious, or simply summoning enough will-power to set things right. "Rejoicing always" will not be easy. Many times, it will require great discipline and personal effort on our part. Depression is a serious problem that requires a serious solution. But by the power of the Holy Spirit, Christians have the resources available to them to overcome this serious problem.

We should note here that "sorrow" is not the same as "depression." In the midst of painful circumstances, there is nothing wrong with a Christian grieving and sorrowing. But in the midst of that pain, we must never be utterly cast down and dejected. We must never become hopeless and pessimistic.

Paul made this point to the Christians in Thessalonica. He wrote to them about the death of their Christian loved ones, saying, "But we do not want you to be uninformed, brethren, about those who are asleep, so that you will not grieve as do the rest who have no hope. For if we believe that Jesus died and rose again, even so God will bring with Him those who have fallen asleep in Jesus…therefore comfort one another with these words" (1 Thessalonians 4:13-14, 18).

Notice that Paul did not rebuke the Thessalonians for their grief. Losing a loved one is a difficult event and it is appropriate for us to sorrow over it. Rather, he reminded them that they were not to grieve as unsaved people grieve—without hope or expectation for the future. Christians should demonstrate appropriate feeling and emotion, but their grief should always be accompanied by great confidence and expectation in the promise of eternal life.

Another passage that illustrates this concept of sorrow accompanied by rejoicing is found in Romans 8:18-39. In these verses Paul wrote about the suffering, trouble, hardship, persecutions, danger and opposition that believers will face in their lives. As we experience these things, Paul said, "…even we ourselves groan within ourselves, waiting eagerly for our adoption as sons, the redemption of our body" (8:23). As believers, we are guaranteed to experience difficult things in our lives that will be painful and sorrowful, but at the same time we are eager and hopeful for what is to come.

In other words, we grieve, but we also have confidence that God is in control of all things. We sorrow, but we also have full assurance that the Spirit of God will help us to be strong and that through Christ we will be more than conquerors in all things. We groan, but we also have a certain and sure conviction that God will work all things together for our good. That is the difference between godly sorrow and sinful depression.

OVERCOMING DEPRESSION CAUSED BY UNBIBLICAL THINKING

In the first chapter, we considered the moderate depression of Asaph (Psalm 73), a psalmist (Psalm 42 and 43), and Jeremiah (Lamentations 3). These four passages not only describe the path these men took to depression, but they also reveal for us eight steps for overcoming depression that is the result of wrong thinking–having unbiblical values, desires, expectations, or standards. In many ways these insights apply to all causes of depression because anyone who refuses to deal with their sin or responds to difficulty in an unbiblical way is obviously not thinking correctly. Therefore we will consider the following eight steps as general principles that apply, to some degree, to all causes of depression:

1. Seek a deeper relationship with God. Psalm 42 begins, "As the deer pants for the water brooks, so my soul pants for You, O God. My soul thirsts for God, for the living God..." (42:1-2). The psalmist demonstrates for us here the first of these eight principles. Ultimately, the only proper and effective way to overcome depression is to be counseled or to counsel oneself in a God-centered way and to actively pursue a more intimate relationship with Him. God must never be an "add-on" or a supplement to the process of overcoming our problems; He must be the very center.

Unfortunately, many people (even believers) do not recognize this. After a seminar in New York, a man came up to me and told me he was a psychotherapist in a local counseling practice. He also said he was a Christian. He went on to explain that when he counseled people, he never introduced the Bible into the counseling discussion because he felt it would be taking unfair advantage of someone in a vulnerable position. "If they tell me they want to talk about God," he continued, "I set up an appointment with them apart from our regular appointments, and there we talk about God and the Bible."

Sadly, many counselors, even those who call themselves Christian take this approach. This kind of counseling advice can also be found in many Christian books and self-help materials on the subject of depression. It is completely unbiblical, however, because it relegates God to a subordinate position. God is simply a supplement to the other, "more relevant," techniques and therapies that are used according to man's wisdom.

We have learned that depression is a problem involving the whole person–physical, emotional, behavioral, intellectual, historical, and most importantly, spiritual. Therefore, a mind and heart that is centered on God is the key to overcoming depression. This is true for two reasons: one, because our spiritual condition is of primary importance in our lives, and two, because of who God is: our Maker and Lord.

71

The writer of Psalms 42 and 43, though he was experiencing a time of depression in his life, was able to keep his focus on God. Consider his words:

"O my God, my soul is in despair within me;
therefore I will remember You from the land of the Jordan, and the peaks of Hermon, from Mount Mizar" (Psalm 42:6).

'The Lord will command His lovingkindness in the daytime; and His song will be with me in the night,
a prayer to the God of my life. I will say to God my rock… ' (Psalm 42:8-9a).

'Vindicate me, O God, and plead my case against an ungodly nation; O deliver me from the deceitful and unjust man! For You are the God of my strength.

O send out your light and Your truth, let them lead me; let them bring me to Your holy hill and to Your dwelling places. Then I will go to the altar of God, to God my exceeding joy; and upon the lyre I shall praise You, O God, my God' (Psalm 43:1-4).

2. Develop open and honest communication with God. Once our focus is squarely on God and we are seeking an increased awareness of His presence in our life, we are on our way to overcoming depression. Again, consider the words of the psalmist:

"O my God, my soul is in despair within me…(Psalm 42:6).
"I will say to God my Rock, 'Why have you forgotten me? Why do I go about mourning because of the oppression of the enemy?'" (Psalm 42:9).

God desires truth at all times, even when our soul is in despair. It is foolish to think that we might fool God by pretending we are fine when we are not because God is all-wise and omniscient. "You understand my thought from afar…Even before there is a word on my tongue, behold, O Lord, You know it all" (Psalm 139:2b, 4). I believe it is appropriate and good for us, even in a time of depression, to be honest about what we are feeling and thinking.

I think it is important, however, to clarify what I mean by honesty with God. I do not believe it is appropriate for us to lash out at God in our anger. Some people have the attitude: "God is big enough to handle it, so I am going to let Him have it!" I believe this attitude is unbiblical because it encourages disrespect toward the One who should have the utmost respect and because it encourages a sinful kind of anger–anger that stems from discontentment and an inadequate understanding of God's character and promises.

While we should never allow ourselves to vent sinful anger against God, it is appropriate to come before God with a submissive spirit and a broken heart. Without charging or blaming God for our problems, we can certainly express to Him our confusion, discouragement, and struggles with the painful circumstances in our lives.

3. We must learn to talk to ourselves rather than listening to ourselves. In fact it is a good idea for all of us, whether we are experiencing depression or not, to make a point of learning this skill and developing it as a habit in our lives. Talking to ourselves can prevent problems in the first place, but listening to ourselves almost always makes problems worse.

What is the danger of listening to ourselves? To listen to ourselves means to freely wander down any path that our mind wishes to take. It is a passive activity that usually results in a constant replaying in the mind of all the unpleasant and painful events and thoughts that have occurred. Each time a hurt is replayed, the memory of it becomes more intense and more painful. Molehills of slights quickly turn into mountains of offense. Eventually, a depressed person will become convinced there is no good in their life at all–that everyone and everything is against them.

On the other hand, when we talk to ourselves, we consciously direct our thoughts in a particular way. After expressing our sadness and hurt to God appropriately, we sit ourselves down and start to ask some hard questions. Consider the psalmist's questioning of himself: "Why are you in despair, O my soul? And why have you become so disturbed within me?" (Psalm 42:5). Three times the psalmist asked himself for a reason for the sadness and despair that he found within his heart (42:5, 11 and 43:5). He deliberately talked to himself, directing his thoughts toward God, "Therefore I remember You..." (Psalm 42:6). This man was not passively accepting the burden of his depression; he was actively seeking to know its cause and to overcome it.

4. We must focus our mind and heart on the facts, not our feelings. Persons who are listening to themselves will be tempted to focus on speculations, assumptions, emotions, and all manner of things based on what is in their heart. As Christians, we ought to know how deceptive our hearts are. Scripture teaches: "The heart is more deceitful than all else and is desperately sick; who can understand it?" (Jeremiah 17:9). Consequently, we must be wary of the lies within it.

Rather than listening to the opinions and lies of our heart, we must focus instead on the truths of God's Word. The psalmist reminded himself, "The Lord *will command* His lovingkindness in the day time; and His song *will be with me* in the night..." (Psalm 42:8). These were facts that the psalmist knew he could count on, and he knew they were true because God said they were true.

In the same way, we must learn to talk to ourselves about the truths that God has revealed to us in His Word. We must meditate daily in the Scripture so that our minds become saturated–soaked–in God's truth. When this becomes our habit, it will replace the natural tendency we all have to passively listen to the deception in our heart.

5. Take charge of our life and realize we are not helpless is the next step to overcoming depression. The psalmist commanded himself, "*Hope in God*, for I shall again praise Him" (42:5, 11; 43:5). As we learned in the previous section, God's children have all the resources they need to overcome at all times and in all things. "And God is able to make *all grace abound to you*, so that *always having all sufficiency in everything*, you may have an abundance for every good deed" (2 Corinthians 9:8).

Though at times we will *feel* helpless, we must again remember that our feelings are deceptive and must not be believed when they run counter to the truth of God's Word. 1 Corinthians 10:13 promises, "*No temptation* has overtaken you but such as is common to man; and *God is faithful, who will not allow you to be tempted beyond what you are able*, but with the temptation will provide the way of escape also, so that you will be able to endure it." We always have a choice between believing the truth of God's Word and believing the lies of the devil.

There are four terrible lies that the devil wants us to believe about our difficulties. The first lie is that we are unique in what we are experiencing. The second lie is that God is not faithful and has forgotten about us. Lie number three is that God is going to test us beyond our ability to endure it. And the fourth lie is that our situation is hopeless and inescapable. 1 Corinthians 10:13 assures us that *none* of these is true.

While it is true that we can do nothing in our own strength, God is more than capable of helping us in all things. "I can do all things through Him who strengthens me" (Philippians 4:13). Though we may *feel weak*, the truth is that we *are strong* in Christ. Thus, we must teach ourselves to move out in faith despite our feelings, believing that God is faithful and that He will help us as He promised.

6. Develop a long-distance view of life. In other words, we need to learn how to look beyond what is happening today and think about the good that God has promised to bring about in the future. At the very end of Psalm 43, the psalmist wrote, "...for I shall again praise Him, the help of my countenance and my God" (43:5). He realized that this was not the end and that he would again be able to praise God because "He is our refuge and strength, a very present help in trouble" (Psalm 46:1).

Joseph is a great example of someone who had a long-distance view of his life. Joseph waited many long years from the time that his brothers sold him into slavery until the time he was Prime Minister of Egypt. He endured many years of trial, persecution, and rejection before God's good purpose was revealed in his life. How many of us would be willing to wait that long to see the good that God had planned for us?

Joseph was able to wait because he read the present in the light of the future, rather than the future in the light of the present. He interpreted his present circumstances through God's promises to him. When he was just a young man, God revealed to him in several dreams that one day all his brothers would bow down to him. Joseph believed that promise and it kept him from despairing through many, many years of trial.

More often, when people experience depression, they do the opposite of what Joseph did. They look at the difficult circumstances of the present and assume that it is always going to be so for them. If they are miserable now, they will surely be miserable always. This is a most unbiblical view of life, and as believers, we must not allow ourselves to think that way.

In 2 Corinthians 4:16, Paul said, "…though our outer man is decaying, yet our inner man is being renewed day by day." The daily renewal of our inner man that Paul wrote about comes by the power of God's Spirit working within us. It also comes by looking, as Paul did, "…not at the things which are seen, but at the things which are not seen; for the things which are seen are temporal, but the things which are not seen are eternal" (4:18). God's promises are eternal and provide for us an accurate and hope-filled, long-distance view of our lives.

7. Learn to be patient. Whether working with someone who is experiencing depression, or counseling ourselves through a time of depression, patience is the key. We must be realistic in our expectations for change. As we have already seen, the psalmist questioned and commanded himself three times:

> "Why are you in despair, O my soul?
> And why have you become disturbed within me?
> Hope in God, for I shall again praise Him,
> the help of my countenance and my God."

As he counseled himself, he probably found that his spirit was lifted a little. Then, he became discouraged again. So he counseled himself some more, was lifted a little, and then discouraged again.

John Bunyan depicted this truth so well in Christian's encounter with Giant Despair. After languishing in the dungeon for some time, Christian reached into his pocket and was surprised to find a key. All the time he and Hopeful had been suffering in the dungeon of the Giant Despair, Christian had forgotten about that key. The key, of course, represents the promises of God that Christian knew, but neglected to remember and meditate on. Using the key, Christian was able to open the dungeon door and go through it.

But depression is never so easily or quickly overcome, as Bunyan wisely knew. No sooner had Christian left the inner room of that dungeon but he found another locked door. Again the key opened it, and again there was another door to be opened. Bit by bit he struggled forward, relapsed into depression, and forced himself onward again. God's promises always worked, but Christian had to reclaim and believe them again and again along the way.

In the same way, we must be prepared to patiently continue to challenge ourselves, or whoever we are counseling, with the truths of God's Word because our minds tend to forget. Moderate or severe depression is not usually overcome in a day, a week, or even a month. It may require endurance through a lengthy period of time.

A mind that is deeply rooted in the negative and that has for so long focused on the lies of the heart and of the devil will not usually become infused with God's truth overnight. We *will* feel badly again. We *will* lose sight of the hope at the end. Struggles, relapses, and temporary failures are all part of overcoming depression. But if we recognize and expect this, we can teach ourselves not to take these set-backs so seriously.

Again, the long-distance view comes into play. While our progress may be slow and sometimes in the wrong direction, by God's grace, *we will make progress*. Knowing this, we can manage the occasional squall instead of thinking that we are going to be swamped by the gathering storm. We can cling to the truth of 2 Corinthians 4:17, "For momentary, light affliction is producing for us an eternal weight of glory far beyond all comparison."

8. Reflect on a holistic view of God. When struggling with depression, we often think about God's justice, holiness, righteousness, and anger. These are important and true aspects of His being, but He is also a God of lovingkindness, mercy and grace, who is long-suffering and forgives.

Instead of selecting certain attributes of God's character that, in a time of depression, cause us to become even more discouraged, we must remind ourselves of *all* of God's attributes. This is the only way we will realize the hope and encouragement He desires for us. The psalmist was no doubt encouraged when he remembered, "The Lord will command His lovingkindness in the daytime..." (Psalm 42:8) and, "Then I will go to the altar of God, to God my exceeding joy…" (Psalm 43:4).

In the same way, we must balance our knowledge of God's holiness with recognition of His mercy. We must counter the truth of His justice and righteousness with the comfort of His grace. We must remember that, although He is justified in His anger against sinful man, He is also "compassionate and gracious, slow to anger and abounding in lovingkindness" (Psalm 103:8). Above all, we must remember that in all things He is *good*, "For You, Lord, are good, and ready to forgive, and abundant in lovingkindness to all who call upon You" (Psalm 86:5).

THE BLESSINGS OF OBEDIENCE

If we faithfully walk in obedience to God's Word, we can be confident that with His help we will overcome depression. This is the path of duty for all of God's children, but it is also the path of delight. Our Lord has promised, "If you know these things, you are blessed if you do them" (John 13:17), and, "…one who looks intently at the perfect law, the law of liberty, and abides by it, not having become a forgetful hearer but an effectual doer, this man will be blessed in what he does" (James 1:25).

Consider the example of a woman who at one time was a living illustration of a severely depressed person. When she came for counseling she was experiencing all of the previously mentioned symptoms of severe depression. Several months after I finished counseling with her, she sent me this letter describing the changes God had made in her life:

Dear Wayne,

I just had to enclose a letter to let you know how well I've been doing. Usually, for the past seven Christmases, I've been terribly depressed during the holiday season. This year, however, my heart is filled with joy for what He has done for me and for Who He is to me. My soul praises Him. I still have some real "downers" occasionally, but even then it is well with my soul and I have an assurance I've never had before.

As I had my devotions the other day, I prayed that God would never let me forget the pain I have suffered and never let me become insensitive, especially to hurting people. Then it occurred to me; it was as though I was almost asking Him to allow the thorn in my side to remain, lest I forget or stop growing. For how could it be humanly possible that I ask for the thorn to remain? It has been so painful to me and I have prayed so long that He take it from me.

I am slowly learning that His grace is sufficient no matter what. I must surely be a slow learner. I think of you and your counseling sessions with me and I thank the Lord for you and the wisdom He gave you, and the receptive heart that He gave me. My inner man is being renewed day by day. Several more people have sought me out for help [depressed friends], just in the past few weeks. I feel as though God is really using me. I'm still witnessing and believing He has made me more useful through my depression, painful as it has been. May you, Carol, and your family have a blessed holiday season.

In the next chapter we will continue to focus our thoughts on this biblical procedure for overcoming depression by examining several examples of depressed people who followed the guidelines for overcoming depression described in this chapter. But before you proceed to that chapter, I again encourage you to spend some time thinking about and answering the following questions:

QUESTIONS FOR DISCUSSION AND APPLICATION:

1. What is the universal requirement for preventing and overcoming depression?

2. What are the necessary steps for preventing or overcoming the depression caused by unresolved personal sin? Twelve steps are listed in this chapter. What are they?

3. Explain what Paul did and didn't mean in Philippians 4:4.

4. What relevance does this statement have to preventing and overcoming depression?

5. What biblical passages help us to understand what Paul meant and didn't mean in Philippians 4:4?

6. To be able to "rejoice in the Lord always" what must we do? What eight principles or steps are laid out in this chapter for doing what Philippians 4:4 exhorts us to do?

7. What are the four terrible lies the devil wants us to believe about our circumstances? (1 Corinthians 10:13)

8. What does developing a long-distance view of life have to do with preventing and overcoming depression?

9. Explain the meaning of the statement that "to prevent and overcome depression we must learn to be patient."

10. What does reflecting on a holistic view of God have to do with preventing and overcoming depression?

11. Carefully reflect on the poem with which this chapter concludes. As you do, answer the questions: What does this poem have to say about what a depressed person is thinking and feeling? What does this poem say about the solution to depression? What helpful perspectives did the person who wrote this poem adopt? What changes took place in her thinking?

12. Have you personally experienced a case of the blues from which you were delivered when you implemented the biblical truths explained in this chapter? Explain the specifics of the situations related to your deliverance from your moderate or severe case of the blues.

13. What have you personally, or for the sake of helping others, learned from this chapter about overcoming depression that will be helpful in your own life or in your ministry to others?

14. Do the things presented in this chapter for overcoming depression make biblical sense? In other words, are they supported by Scripture?

Chapter 5
Getting Out of the Blues- Biblical Examples

The eight key principles, in whole or in part, for overcoming the kind of depression that is caused by mishandling a difficult situation or by adopting an unbiblical value system may be found in many places in Scripture. In this chapter we will look at the examples of how Asaph, Jeremiah and David overcame depression by putting these principles into practice. They counseled themselves with biblical truth.

ASAPH'S EXAMPLE

In Psalm 77 Asaph began, "My voice rises to God, and I will cry aloud; my voice rises to God, and He will hear me" (77:1). From the very beginning of Asaph's account of his struggle with depression, we see that Asaph had his focus on God. He was crying out to God for help in this time of difficulty, which he went on to describe:

> In the day of trouble I sought the Lord;
> In the night my hand was stretched out without weariness;
> My soul refused to be comforted.
> When I remember God, then I am disturbed;
> When I sigh, then my spirit grows faint.
> You have held my eyelids open;
> I am so troubled that I cannot speak (Psalm 77:2-4).

We see in these verses that Asaph freely and honestly admitted his struggle to God. He knew that his relationship with God was not right, which is very common in a time of depression.

As we learned in the last chapter, depression is usually the result of one of three things: refusing to deal with sin and guilt, mishandling a difficult event, or having unbiblical standards. These three problems can only occur when there is a problem in one's relationship with God. As a result, when someone is in the midst of depression, they often do not want to discuss God or biblical things because they sense the underlying problem in their heart. When they think about God, it bothers them as it did Asaph. Asaph admitted his struggle and then continued to be open and honest with God about how he felt:

> I have considered the days of old,
> The years of long ago.
> I will remember my song in the night;
> I will meditate with my heart,
> And my spirit ponders:
> Will the Lord reject forever?
> And will He never be favorable again?
> Has His lovingkindness ceased forever?
> Has His promise come to an end forever?
> Has God forgotten to be gracious,
> Or has He in anger withdrawn His compassion?
> Then I said, "It is my grief,
> That the right hand of the Most High has changed"
> (Psalm 77:5-10).

What honesty this man had in his heart before God! Notice, however, that his honesty was respectful and never accusing. He never shook his fist at God.

Then after pouring out his heart to God, the psalmist dramatically took charge of himself and began to talk to his spirit instead of listening to it. He focused his thoughts on the truths that he knew about God:

> I shall remember the deeds of the Lord;
> Surely I will remember Your wonders of old.
> I will meditate on all Your work
> And muse on Your deeds.
> Your way, O God, is holy;
> What god is great like our God?
> You are the God who works wonders;

You have made known Your strength among the
peoples.
You have by Your power redeemed Your people,
The sons of Jacob and Joseph. (Psalm 77:11-15).

Asaph stopped exchanging the truth of God for a lie (Romans 1:25)
and set His mind on what he knew about God; that God does not reject
or forget His children (Deuteronomy 31:8), that His lovingkindness
never ceases (Deuteronomy 7:9), that God is holy (Leviticus 11:44),
and that God saves those who call out to Him (2 Samuel 22:2-51).

And Asaph continued to direct his thoughts according to what He
knew about God:

The waters saw You, O God;
The waters saw You, they were in anguish;
The deeps also trembled.
The clouds poured out water;
The skies gave forth a sound;
Your arrows flashed here and there.
The sound of Your thunder was in the whirlwind;
The lightnings lit up the world;
The earth trembled and shook.
Your way was in the sea
And Your paths in the mighty water,
And Your footprints may not be known.
You led Your people like a flock
By the hand of Moses and Aaron. (Psalm 77:16-20).

Asaph remembered what he knew about God, and as he looked
around him at creation, Asaph refocused his mind on God's awesome
power.

God's power should be a tremendous encouragement to us. When
we think about what God can do, what God does do, and what God
promises to do for us, we should be encouraged and filled with hope.
"...He does according to His will in the host of Heaven and among
the inhabitants of the earth; and no one can ward off His hand or say
to Him, 'What have You done?'" (Daniel 4:35).

JEREMIAH'S EXAMPLE

Jeremiah also experienced a time of depression. His discouragement and the way in which he counseled himself during this time are recorded for us in Lamentations. After honestly describing how he felt, Jeremiah directed his thoughts to God: "Remember my affliction and my wandering, the wormwood and bitterness" (3:19). Then he began to talk to himself:

> This I recall to mind,
> Therefore I have hope.
> The Lord's lovingkindnesses indeed never cease,
> For His compassions never fail.
> They are new every morning;
> Great is Your faithfulness.
> "The Lord is my portion," says my soul,
> "Therefore I have hope in Him" (Lamentations 3:21-24).

Jeremiah forced himself to think about what he knew of God's character: His lovingkindness, compassion, faithfulness, and provision. He meditated on these things because they gave him hope.

After reflecting on some facts about God's character, Jeremiah took charge of his mind and reflected on the fact that God had a purpose for the adversity that He allowed into his life:

> The Lord is good to those who wait for Him,
> To the person who seeks Him.
> It is good that he waits silently
> For the salvation of the Lord.
> It is good for a man that he should bear
> The yoke in his youth.
> Let him sit alone and be silent
> Since He has laid it on him.
> Let him put his mouth in the dust,
> Perhaps there is hope.
> Let him give his cheek to the smiter,
> Let him be filled with reproach (Lamentations 3:25-30).

Jeremiah clearly had the ABC view of life: Adversity Builds Character. In light of this, he admonished his soul to do three things.

First, he told himself to be silent before God and not to argue and protest his affliction (3:28). Next, he told himself to be humble before God and realize that God brings trials to teach and strengthen, not to crush or punish (27-29). Then he told himself to have meekness toward men because kindness turns away anger (Proverbs 15:1). Finally Jeremiah decided to take a long-distance view of his suffering and be patient for God's timing:

> For the Lord will not reject forever,
> For if He causes grief,
> Then He will have compassion
> According to His abundant lovingkindness.
> For He does not afflict willingly
> Or grieve the sons of men.
> To crush under His feet
> All the prisoners of the land,
> To deprive a man of justice
> In the presence of the Most High,
> To defraud a man in his lawsuit—
> Of these things the Lord does not approve.
> Who is there who speaks and it comes to pass,
> Unless the Lord has commanded it?
> Is it not from the mouth of the Most High
> That both good and ill go forth? (Lamentations 3:31-38).

Jeremiah thought about the fact that God was in control of everything in his life and that God disciplines those whom He loves (Hebrews 12:5-6), doing it "unwillingly," as a father disciplines his son.

As a father, I found no joy in spanking my children. When I spanked them, it was for their benefit. While the child always finds it hard to believe that "this hurts me more than it does you," a parent knows how true that statement is. "For [our earthly fathers] disciplined us for a short time as seemed best to them, but He disciplines us for our good, so that we may share His holiness" (Hebrews 12:10).

God does not afflict us because He enjoys making us miserable. On the contrary, God desires only to bless us. But sometimes, the best kind of blessing that we can receive is a trial that will make us stronger and more Christ-like in our character. "All discipline for the moment seems not to be joyful, but sorrowful; yet to those who have been trained by it, afterwards it yields the peaceful fruit of righteousness" (Hebrews 12:11).

DAVID'S EXAMPLE

We have already looked at several examples of times in David's life when he struggled with depression, most notably after refusing to deal with his sin of adultery. But even a casual study of David's life from Scripture demonstrates that it was not characterized by depression. Why was this true despite numerous difficulties? David was not defeated by depression because he wisely refused to focus his mind on his problems or his feelings and instead firmly resolved to fix his mind on God. On the whole, he looked at life through God's eyes and analyzed and approached every situation through the promises and person of God.

That is not to say that David was a dreamer or a fool who simply looked at the world through rose-colored glasses. David faced difficult situations in his life and had problems that could have, and occasionally did, drive him to despair; persecution from King Saul, rejection by his son, severe punishment by God for his sin of adultery, among other things. But by and large he refused to look at his life without first looking at God. He knew that "the steps of a man are established by the Lord..." (Psalm 37:23). He knew that his Heavenly Father loved him and would turn tragedy into triumph, problems into progress, burdens into blessings, and stumbling blocks into stepping stones.

Consequently, David was able to go through most of his life with God in focus. He was able to overcome the temptation to despondency by talking to himself, preaching to himself, exhorting himself, and encouraging himself in the Lord. Certainly there were times when he failed in this, and on those occasions, he struggled with a time of despondency. But he always regained his focus, and, as a result could say, "The lines have fallen to me in pleasant places; indeed my heritage is beautiful to me...my heart is glad, and my glory [inner self] rejoices; my flesh will also dwell securely" (Psalm 16:6, 9, explanation added).

RUNNING THE RACE WITH ENDURANCE

In looking at these few, relatively short passages, we must not be fooled into thinking that the problem of depression can be easily or quickly overcome. Anyone who has experienced depression knows that it can be deeply ingrained in one's life and *often* requires a long and diligent effort to overcome.

Psalms 42 and 43 seem to indicate that overcoming depression is much more of a process than an event. It would appear from these passages that the writer's depression developed and continued over an extended period of time. It also seems likely from what is written that the psalmist made some measure of progress a number of times, but then his depression would return. In Lamentations we see that Jeremiah had to learn to "wait silently," indicating that his depression and its resolution were a lengthy process.

I remember a woman I counseled for depression some years ago. She had struggled with depression for at least thirty years of her life, and had been unsuccessfully "treated" by various "mental health experts." When she first came to me, she had just tried to commit suicide, had been hospitalized for a time, and had almost been forced to come to my office. By that point, she had basically given up on her life; she did no housework, never went to church, and rarely even got out of bed in the morning.

As we worked together, she made very slow progress at first, but she stuck with it. And by God's grace, she began to change bit by bit despite her initial doubts. Though it took several months of counseling and much perseverance on her part, eventually she came to a place where she did not need counseling anymore. Several months after we stopped meeting together, she wrote me a letter thanking me for helping her, and praising God for His goodness to her.

The process of being delivered from depression may follow the course described in the following diagrams. In the Stage 1 phase, the depressed person is looking primarily at the difficult circumstances he is encountering **without serious thoughts about God's involvement**. At this point, thoughts about God are largely being blocked out by thoughts about the immensity and difficulty of the circumstances. If he thinks about God's relationship to his problems at all, he does so in a very superficial manner. For him, God is small, insignificant, and irrelevant, and the circumstances and obstacles are enormous, overwhelming, and insurmountable.

Stage 1

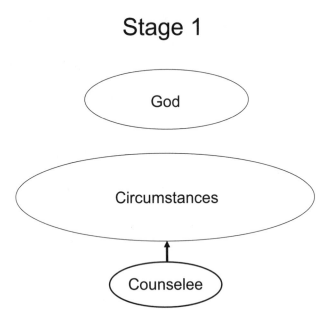

In the Stage 2 phase of the process of overcoming depression, **God is brought into the picture.** Because of his reading or what he hears in a sermon, or because of the efforts of a godly counselor, the depressed person begins to think about God's involvement in what is happening. At this phase of the process of overcoming depression, the depressed person tends to read and think about God through the lens of his circumstances. He understands that somehow God is involved in what is happening, but the circumstances seem much larger than God can or will handle. As he thinks about his difficulties, he is perplexed by the thought that if God is involved in what is happening, and if God is really a God of love, wisdom and power, He would not have allowed things such as these to occur, or he would be doing something to remove them. His own mind, not God's Word, is the standard by which he interprets the character of God and the nature of his own circumstances. The result is that his depression, except for possible brief periods of relief, continues to dominate his life.

Stage 2

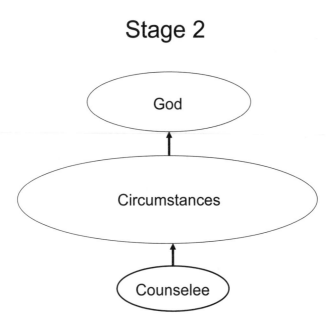

In the Stage 3 phase of the process of overcoming depression, **the attitude and perspective of the depressed person begins to change because he disciplines himself to focus on the Bible's interpretation, rather than his own or the world's interpretation,** of God and the situation. As he faithfully and consistently allows the Word of Christ to richly dwell in him (Colossians 3:16), the Holy Spirit helps Him to think biblically about the character of God and his situation. As he meditates and delights in God's Word (Psalm 1:1-3), he stops interpreting God through his circumstances and begins to understand who and what God is through the Living Word (Jesus Christ) and the written Word (the Bible). Gradually the Holy Spirit delivers him from being conformed to the world's perspective on the immensity, hopelessness and uselessness of his difficulties and, by the aid of the Holy Spirit, he begins to view what is happening in his life from God's perspective.

Instead of viewing God through his circumstances, he begins to view his circumstances through the eyes of God, as God interprets them in His Word. Instead of thinking merely of the awfulness of the unpleasant things that are happening around him or to him, he begins to accept and be controlled by the truth that God is present and somehow "working all things together for good" (Romans 8:28) and that God is using the circumstances to test and strengthen his faith and make him perfect and complete, "lacking in nothing" (James 1:2-4). As he presses on, knowing and claiming the promises of God, he is encouraged by the reality that he has nothing to fear or be dismayed about because his trustworthy God will most certainly help, strengthen and uphold him with His powerful right hand (Isaiah 41:10). Returning again and again to the biblical fact that if God is for him, who or what can be really against him (Romans 8:31), he is moved upward out of the downward descent into depression.

Stage 3

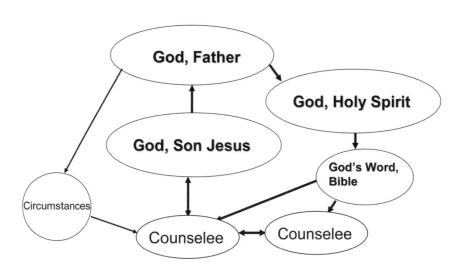

Moving from the situation as depicted in Stage 1 to the situation described in Stage 3 is usually a process that may take a period of time. Though we are often in a hurry to resolve our problems, God's timetable is much different than ours. Sanctification is a life-long process for all believers. Our salvation in Christ has a definite beginning, but there is a sense in which it never has an end on this earth. We are always becoming more and more like Christ, and a large part of that process is struggling to overcome sin in our life. Since God is patient with us, we must also be patient with ourselves.

In Yosemite National Park, two imposing mountains are favorites of serious rock-climbers: El Capitan and Half Dome. Though I cannot imagine doing it myself, I have been told that these climbers must persevere for many days when attempting a complete ascent of these rock walls. After each long day's climb, they drive pitons into the rock, hang a bivouac sack on them, and spend the night dangling over hundreds, even thousands, of feet of air.

As the climbers move upward, winds buffet them, equipment sometimes fails and causes setbacks, sleep is difficult and short, food is cold and merely functional, and the rough rock wall punishes the climber's legs, arms, feet and hands. On top of the constant physical strain, there is the constant mental strain of the fatigue and the fear of failure.

Why do they do it? Why do they put themselves through the almost guaranteed difficulty of a major climb? They do it for the anticipated reward of reaching the top. At the top, there is the satisfaction of an amazing accomplishment and a chance to rest on level ground–not to mention an incredible view.

Overcoming our sin problems is sometimes like climbing a mountain. It involves blood, sweat, and tears. It takes a long time. There are discouraging setbacks along the way. It is physically, mentally, and emotionally exhausting. There are times when it may seem as if we will never make it at all. But like the climbers, we must keep the end always in sight because the reward for overcoming sin is far greater than the reward for reaching the top of a mountain. We have much, much more to look forward to when we finally overcome!

So how do we keep ourselves going when the end is still so far away and our present progress is so very slow? As we learned earlier, we must have a Philippians 4:13 attitude: "I can do all things through Him who strengthens me." We must remember first that we can do nothing on our own. Anything that is accomplished in us is by the grace of God and the power of His Holy Spirit in us. Second, we must not believe the lie of our unbelieving hearts that says, "I can't do it anymore. It's just too hard." Instead, we must remind ourselves that we can do all things with God's help.

This is what it means to live by faith and not by sight. In the midst of depression, the road may seem very dark and the storm may feel very strong, but God has not asked us to live by what we can see or feel. We must have faith that God is the source of all light and our refuge from the storm. We must continue walking as He has commanded us to, knowing that, "Even the darkness is not dark to You" (Psalm 139:12), and that "even the wind and the sea obey Him!" (Mark 4:41).

Consider again the great truths written by Jeremiah in
Lamentations 3:21-25:
This I recall to my mind,
Therefore I have hope.
The Lord's lovingkindnesses indeed never cease,
For His compassions never fail.
They are new every morning;
Great is Your faithfulness.
"The Lord is my portion," says my soul,
"Therefore I have hope in Him."
The Lord is good to those who wait for Him,
To the person who seeks Him.

May the Lord, in His goodness, call these things continually to our minds so that we may walk by faith in His promises and not in sight of our circumstance. And now before moving on to the next chapter I encourage you to complete the following application exercises. Purchase a small notebook and write the assignments in one location for frequent reference.

APPLICATION EXERCISES:

1. Make a list of the biblical principles for overcoming depression that were discussed in the last two chapters. Put a check mark in front of the principles on this list which you are guilty of violating. Specifically confess your failure to God, seek cleansing through the blood of Christ, and ask for the help of the Holy Spirit to become more biblical in the way that you handle the temptation to depression.

2. Ask other people to pray for you and to exhort you to biblical obedience. Stay away from people who give you the wrong kind of sympathy and encourage you in your self-pity, excuse-making, brooding, or neglect of your responsibilities. Study 1 Corinthians 15:33; Proverbs 22:24-25, 14:7; Galatians 6:1; Hebrews 3:12-13 and 10:24-25 concerning the kinds of companions you need. Decide whom you will ask for prayer and encouragement and ask them.

3. Make a "think and do" list of profitable things you can think about and do when you are tempted to be depressed. Use Philippians 4:8-9 to help you in this. Keep this list with you on a 3 x 5 card; pull it out and use it when you begin to feel depressed.

4. Make a list of your responsibilities. Note which ones you are fulfilling well and regularly. Also note those you have been neglecting, or are prone to neglect, because you don't feel like doing them. Ask God to help you do what you should, regardless of how you feel. Plan a schedule that gives you time to do all that you really must do and then get busy fulfilling your responsibilities. Don't focus on how badly you feel or how much you dislike a particular task. Focus rather on God, His will for you, His promises and provisions for you, and the help He will give you to do anything He wants you to do (Philippians 2:12-13; 4:13).

5. Make a list of at least fifty to seventy-five blessings that God has bestowed on you. Think about every area of your life: spiritual, physical, financial, social, circumstantial, mental, relational, etc. Continue to add to this list as you become aware of new benefits God is bestowing on you, remembering that Psalm 68:19 says that He daily loads us with benefits. As you make your list of benefits, specifically thank God for each of them. Make it a daily practice to give specific thanks for specific things (Philippians 4:8; Psalm 34:1; Ephesians 5:20).

6. Make a list of some of the hard and challenging things in your life. By faith and in obedience to God's Word (Ephesians 5:20; 1 Thessalonians 5:18; James 1:2-4), give thanks to God for what He is going to do in you and through you because of these things. Give thanks for the help He is going to give you and for using these things to teach you discipline, or to cause you to examine your life, or to remind you of sins, etc.

7. Study Job 23:10; Romans 5:1-4, Romans 8:14-29; James 1:2-4, Philippians 1:12-19; Psalm 34:1-4; Psalm 76:10; Isaiah 50:10; 2 Corinthians 12:7-10; Hebrews 12:1-15; Proverbs 15:13, 15; Psalm 119:67, 71; Job 5:17-18; 2 Corinthians 1:3-11; and 1 Peter 1:6-7 and write down everything these passages teach us about God's purpose for hardships, how we should respond to them, and

what God can do through them. Review the results of your study whenever you are tempted to be depressed and specifically thank God for His help to overcome this temptation.

8. Establish a regular practice of daily Bible reading and study, prayer and meditation. Plan your procedure of study, schedule a regular time for your devotions, and put your plans into action. Keep a written record of what you learn in your devotional time. Ask mature Christians for help in making them more profitable. Seek immediately to implement what you learn and to share it with other people.

9. Make a list of specific ways that you are failing God, your family, your employer, your church, your neighbor, etc. Confess your sins to God and ask for forgiveness. Seek His help to change and get busy becoming the kind of person God wants you to be. If your sin has specifically and publicly involved other people, ask them for forgiveness. The sphere of your confession should be as broad as the sphere of people who have knowingly been hurt by your sin (Matthew 5:21-26). When confessing sin, be brief and to the point and beware of violating the principles laid down in Ephesians 5:1-6, Matthew 7:1-5, and James 4:11.

10. Get a copy of **A Christian Growth and Discipleship Manual** by Wayne Mack and Wayne Johnston and do some of the assignments in the second section of the book, which is the hope-giving section. Focus especially on the studies on God's love, God as our Father, the resources we have in Christ, and the studies on the life of Joseph and Paul. The book, **Down But Not Out** by Wayne Mack will also be a helpful reading assignment.

Finally, seek out a biblical counselor and ask them to help you become more biblical in your lifestyle in general, and in overcoming depression in particular. Your main desire in life should be to glorify God, and that will only happen as you become more biblical in your living and thinking. If you have not been able to overcome depression on your own, plan now to seek help from a godly counselor. Make the effort to contact this person and set up an appointment to meet with them as soon as possible.

Chapter 6
Loneliness or Lonely-less?

There is an old gospel song that says, "On life's pathway I am never lonely, my Lord is with me, my Lord divine." The chorus continues, "No longer lonely, no longer lonely, for my Lord is with me, my Lord divine." It's a beautiful song with lovely words and melody, but I am convinced that few, if any, people can honestly sing it. Perhaps a few can say, "On life's pathway I am *seldom* lonely," but very few people can honestly say, "On life's pathway I am *never* lonely."

Loneliness: A Common Experience

The truth of the matter is that loneliness is a very common experience. It is felt by both young and old, rich and poor, unbeliever and believer alike. Most of us, at some point, can identify with the words of David in Psalm 142: "Look to the right and see; for there is no one who regards me; there is no escape for me; no one cares for my soul." (142:4). He pleaded with God for relief from his loneliness as he went on, "Give heed to my cry, for I am brought very low;... bring my soul out of prison" (142:6-7a).

Most of us probably know of someone who is struggling with loneliness. I know of a lady who lives all alone and because of that, she never does her grocery shopping at a large supermarket. Instead, she goes every day to a little corner store just so that she can have some daily contact with other people.

I know of another woman who lived alone in Philadelphia, Pennsylvania. One day her neighbors noticed that she was no longer coming and going as she usually did, so they called the police. The police broke in and found her alive but very sick. She was taken to the hospital, where she eventually recovered. But as she was preparing to return home, a policeman came by the hospital and told her that they needed to exterminate the rats and mice in her apartment before she could go back. To his surprise, the woman begged him not to have this done because, she said, "They're the only friends I have." There are lonely people all around us, and we may never be aware of them.

Loneliness: A Painful Experience

Loneliness is a very common experience, but it is also a very painful and unpleasant one. In 1 Kings 19 the prophet Elijah was greatly distressed; so distressed that he asked God to take his life. Being a child of God, he would never have committed suicide, but he so wanted to die that he asked God to take his life away. Two times in this passage Elijah told the Lord, "I alone am left." In the context of the events taking place at that time, it is clear as we noted in previous chapters that one of the reasons Elijah wanted to die was because he felt so miserably depressed. Undoubtedly his loneliness was a facilitating factor in the depression he experienced.

The Lord Jesus experienced painful loneliness in the Garden of Gethsemane. Near the end of His life on earth, He brought three of His disciples with Him to the garden and asked them to keep watch with Him. He knew that the time was quickly approaching when He would have to face the agony of the cross, so He asked His three most intimate disciples to stay up and pray with Him. As we know from Scripture, His disciples went to sleep instead.

And surely none of us has experienced the excruciating loneliness that Christ must have felt as He hung on the cross. The Scripture says that God the Father poured out His wrath for our sins on Christ. As noonday light turned to darkness, Jesus cried out, "My God, My God, why have You forsaken Me?" (Mark 15:33-34). I believe that one of the most painful aspects of the crucifixion was the terrible loneliness that Christ must have felt on the cross, bearing the sins of His people and the wrath of His Father.

The apostle Paul knew loneliness to be a painful experience. In 2 Timothy 4, he told Timothy to "*make every effort* to come to me soon" (4:9). In the next few verses, Paul explained why he so longed for Timothy to come, "...for Demas, having loved this present world, has deserted me...Crescens has gone to Galatia, Titus to Dalmatia. Only Luke is with me..." (10-11). Paul was virtually alone and eager for Timothy's company.

Loneliness is just as painful today as it was long ago. One fourteen year-old girl described the pain of loneliness this way: "As I write this note my hand is shaking, my eyes are full of tears, and my heart is aching. I am so lonely." An older man, a seminary professor, who was struggling with loneliness said, "It feels as if there is a big hole in the middle of my chest. Sometimes it's a dull pain–a listlessness. Everything is tasteless; even that which I most enjoy seems pointless, even painful, because I respond to it by wanting to share it. But when I reach out to do so, there is no one there. I feel cut off, empty, isolated from the others I need." Loneliness is indeed a painful and distressing experience.

Loneliness: A Destructful Experience

Loneliness can also be a very destructive experience. It seldom visits alone, usually bringing with it any number of evil friends– depression, anger, doubt, guilt, self-pity, or anxiety. Inevitably, these evil friends lock arms and strengthen each other in their destructive work.

This happens because a lonely person often becomes angry at his situation, and as a result, becomes lonelier. He feels sorry for himself and becomes even lonelier. The downward spiral continues, with anger giving birth to depression, depression to more anger, and all of these to guilt. Guilt often leads to anxiety and soon enough, destruction is knocking at the door as his problems grow and his soul becomes overwhelmed.

Loneliness: A Problem With A Solution

Loneliness is a common, painful, and often destructive experience. It is not, however, an insurmountable experience. The good news is that help and hope are available to us from God and through His Word. To help us understand how God wants us to handle the problem of loneliness, we need to answer two important questions. First, what are the causes of loneliness? And second, how does God want us to deal with the problem of loneliness?

The Causes of Loneliness

1. A Deficient Relationship with God

One cause of loneliness is a deficient relationship with God. Some people are lonely because they have no relationship with God at all. Isaiah 57:20 says, "But the wicked are like the tossing sea, for it cannot be quiet..." There is restlessness and emptiness in those who do not know God, and that describes anyone who is unsaved. Ephesians 2:12

says, "...remember that you were at that time separate from Christ... having no hope and without God in the world." St. Augustine once said, "Lord you have made us for yourself and our souls are restless until they rest in Thee." Whether they know it or not, the emptiness and loneliness that unbelievers experience are direct results of their separation from God.

While some people are lonely because they have *no* relationship with God, others experience loneliness because they are *neglecting* their relationship with God. These are people who have been brought to repentance and faith by the Holy Spirit, but have not progressed in their faith.

The Scripture says that, as believers, we must "walk as children of Light (for the fruit of the Light consists in all goodness and righteousness and truth), trying to learn what is pleasing to the Lord" (Ephesians 5:8-10). In other words, we must walk in obedience, living a life that is according to the will of God, in order to have a proper and growing fellowship with the Father. Many believers are lonely because they are not walking in obedience.

Jesus taught this when He said, "If anyone loves Me, he will keep My word; and My Father will love him, and We will come to him and make Our abode with him" (John 14:23). We must keep God's word–His commandments–in order to receive spiritual insight and experience the close fellowship of God the Father. God reveals Himself and dwells with those who obey Him. Some Christians experience deep loneliness because they neglect their relationship with God.

2. The Transient Nature of Life

Some people experience loneliness because of the transient nature of life. The psalmist wrote about the frailty of life: "As for man, his days are like grass; as a flower of the field, so he flourishes. When the wind has passed over it, it is no more, and its place acknowledges it no longer" (Psalm 103:15-16). James 4:14 says, "...you do not know what your life will be like tomorrow. You are just a vapor that appears for a little while and then vanishes away."

Life is indeed transitory and frail and because of this, we cannot completely avoid loneliness. People die, move away, or change jobs and this means that relationships are constantly changing; sometimes ending. These things bring on an understandable and expected sense of loss and emptiness. We feel lonely when our best friend moves far away, when a trusted co-worker finds a new job, or when a family member dies and we know that we will never see them again in this world.

Relationships among believers are affected as people move from church to church. When I've had the opportunity to visit some churches I once pastored, I have often noticed a nearly complete turnover in the membership. In terms of the relationships in our lives, we live in a constant state of flux, and that means some amount of loneliness is inevitable.

3. The Nature of our Responsibilities

Loneliness is sometimes caused by the nature of our responsibilities and commitments. Elijah was lonely, to some extent, because of his responsibilities. In 1 Kings 18, the Scripture says that God sent Elijah to the top of Mount Carmel where he alone challenged the people of Israel, saying, "How long will you hesitate between two opinions? If the Lord is God, follow Him; but if Baal, follow him…I alone am left a prophet of the Lord" (18:21-22). He then challenged the 450 prophets of Baal and 400 prophets of Asherah to a contest to call down rain from Heaven. Elijah was clearly submissive to God and, as a result, had weighty responsibilities. Because of this, he was not able to be among the people as much and had many enemies as well.

The same was true of Paul. Paul preached the gospel and was steadfastly committed to the truth of God's Word. Though many people appreciated Paul and his ministry, there were plenty of people who did not. And those who did not would do anything to stop him. They threw him out of town, stoned him, and put him in prison. Paul experienced times of loneliness because of his commitment to the gospel and to serving Jesus Christ.

As we mentioned earlier, our Lord Jesus Christ experienced loneliness as well because of His commitment to God the Father. People hated Him because of who He was and because He convicted them of their sin. We may be sure that as believers, we will experience some loneliness because of our commitment to Jesus Christ. In John 15:18, Jesus warned, "If the world hates you, you know that it has hated Me before it hated you."

1 John 3:1 says, "See how great a love the Father has bestowed on us…for this reason the world does not know us, because it did

not know Him." In other words, the world will reject us because it rejected Christ, and we cannot escape it. If we stand up for the truth of God's Word and preach the gospel, we will cause offense and we will be rejected, ridiculed, and isolated because of it. Believers will surely experience loneliness because of their commitment to Christ and their responsibility to serve Him.

4. Our Sins and Failures

Loneliness is sometimes caused by our sins and failures. While there is nothing we can do about the transient nature of life or being rejected by others because of our faith, we are certainly to blame for the loneliness that results from our sins and failures. And there are numerous sins that can lead to loneliness.

Some people are lonely because they are fearful. They are afraid to reach out, afraid to try to develop relationships with other people, because they do not want to be rejected. I know of a young man who, for months, would not ask a young lady out on a date because he was afraid he would be rejected. He was so afraid of rejection that he preferred to not have a date at all rather than to ask for a date and be turned down. There are many other people who refuse to reach out to others because they are afraid that their efforts will be wasted or their feelings hurt.

Others are afraid of being taken advantage of. They don't want to be in a position where they are being asked to give more than they are receiving in the relationship, so they stay a safe distance away from other people. In reality, this is selfishness. 1 John 4:18 says, "There is no fear in love; but perfect love casts out fear…" In other words, if we have fear, it is because we do not have love.

Fearful people are always thinking about themselves: "What are they going to think of me?" They are wrapped up in their own concerns, wondering what might happen to them. But love never thinks about self; love thinks only about the other person: "How can I serve this person? What do they need?" Love has no fear because fear is inward-oriented thinking and love is entirely outward-oriented thinking.

For example, I do quite a bit of preaching and teaching on topics related to thinking and living biblically. If I were fearful about this, I would worry that people would be bored by my material, or that people would criticize me, or that I would never be invited back. But if instead, I think in love–that God has given me an important message from His Word and that people need to hear it–then I will be bold in my preaching, eager to show love to others by reaching out to them with what they need. Selfish fear is a sin that can lead to loneliness.

In a similar vein, preoccupation with self is a sin that can lead to loneliness. Some people are so focused on themselves that they have difficulty developing real friendships. When other people are around them, all they can do is talk about themselves. Whether it's their talents and successes or their problems and failures, it's all about them. And eventually, many people just stay away from them.

Sometimes people experience loneliness because they fail to open up to other people. They keep everything to themselves, closely guarding the secret matters of their hearts. I have counseled a number of people who were experiencing loneliness, and as I worked with them I was amazed at how many of them were very secretive people. They did not trust others and refused to open themselves up to anyone.

John 1:7 says, "But if we walk in the Light as He Himself is in the Light, we have fellowship with one another, and the blood of Jesus His Son cleanses us from all sin." One of the things that "walking in the light" means is to live transparently–openly and honestly–before others. In other words, we do not try to pretend to be someone or something that we are not; we do not try to cover up our weaknesses. When we walk in the light, we willingly expose ourselves to others and let them see us for who we really are. The Scripture says that this is the key to good relationships with other people–to having "fellowship with one another."

The same is true in terms of our relationship with the Lord. The next two verses go on to say, "If we say that we have no sin, we are deceiving ourselves and the truth is not in us. If we confess our sins, He is faithful and righteous to forgive us our sins and to cleanse us from all unrighteousness" (1 John 1:8-9). Openness and honesty is an absolute requirement for fellowship with God. It is only when we openly admit our sinfulness to God that He forgives us and restores us to a right relationship with Himself.

Walking in the light–being open and honest with God and with other people–is the key to good fellowship. Some time ago, I taught at a Sunday school convention in the Allentown, Pennsylvania area. When I finished teaching, a woman came up to me and said, "I want the in-depth kind of fellowship and friendship with others that you've been talking about. But I don't know anyone who is willing to be open with me. What do I do? I want to be able to go to people for help and to share my problems. I want to be able to help others, but people won't open up." My answer to her was that she had to be the one to start.

Many people are lonely because they never open up to other people. Whether they are failing to take the initiative in this or simply refusing to reciprocate doesn't really matter. The Bible says that we have to be open with each other in order to have fellowship. We cannot truly know another person and have a deep, meaningful friendship unless that person reveals their true self to us and we reveal our true self to them. This means that you may be allowing yourself to be vulnerable to that person, but doing so will begin to build trust, which is a strong basis for friendship.

There are many other sins and failures that can lead to loneliness, but these are an important and common few.

God's Solution To The Problem Of Loneliness

Step 1: Accept the Unavoidable

Now that we know some of the causes of loneliness, we can begin to look at the proper response to this problem. The first step in dealing with loneliness is to *realize and accept the fact that some loneliness is unavoidable*. As we discussed earlier, there are at least two causes of loneliness that are completely out of our hand; the transient nature of life and the nature of some of our responsibilities.

Jesus warned us in John 16:33 that in this world we would experience troubles. In James 1:2, we are told to "consider it all joy, my brethren, *when* you encounter various trials." If any Christian thinks they are going to escape loneliness in this world, they will be very disappointed. But as believers we do have hope in this promised difficulty: "But now, thus says the Lord, your Creator... 'Do not fear, for I have redeemed you...When you pass through the waters, I will be with you; and through the rivers, they will not overflow you. When you walk through the fire, you will not be scorched, nor will the flame burn you'" (Isaiah 43:1-2). Again, we see the word "when" used, indicating that trials should be expected. Loneliness in this present evil world is unavoidable. Some of us will experience much loneliness, others will experience less, but we all will experience some amount of loneliness.

Several years ago, my wife had the opportunity to counsel a woman who had recently lost her husband of some fifty years. Her husband was a wonderful man and they had enjoyed a good relationship. Loneliness was an unavoidable consequence of that loss because suddenly the man that she had shared everything with for fifty years was gone. My wife counseled this woman and gave her some very practical suggestions about what she should do to deal with her loneliness. And though these things certainly helped, quite a while later the woman said to Carol, "I am still experiencing some loneliness." My wife responded, "You're going to have to learn to live with some loneliness; you'll never completely escape it." This is very true, and until we come to the point where we can accept that, we will bring additional pain and unhappiness on ourselves by thinking that we can somehow escape loneliness entirely.

Step 2: Rejoice in the Benefits

The second step to overcoming loneliness is *to recognize that some loneliness may be a beneficial experience.* James 1 continues, "Consider it all joy, my brethren, when you encounter various trials, knowing that the testing of your faith produces endurance. And let endurance have its perfect result, so that you may be perfect and complete, lacking in nothing" (1:2-4). James' message to believers was that trials are indeed painful, but we should be encouraged by the knowledge that God is using them to do good things in our lives. Therefore, we can accept a trial like loneliness as necessary and beneficial.

How can God use loneliness for good in our lives? For one thing, loneliness can stimulate us to greater prayer. In Psalm 142, David cried out to God in his time of loneliness: "I cry aloud with my voice to the Lord; I make supplication with my voice to the Lord" (142:1). If loneliness drives us to God, then that is certainly a good result.

Loneliness can also encourage meditation and reflection. It may cause us to come back to the Word of God as we seek to find out what God has to say about our problem. Loneliness may cause us to examine ourselves, to think about changes we need to make in our lives. These are all beneficial results.

Loneliness may help us to develop understanding and compassion for others in similar situations. It may cause us to realize our need for other people. At times we can become quite independent and not realize, until something happens, how lonely we really are. We need meaningful relationships with other people so we can minister to them and allow them to minister to us as well. If we realize this, loneliness can actually push us to reach out to other people. Though the circumstance of loneliness may be painful, it can help us to improve our relationships with other people.

Finally, loneliness can be beneficial because it can cause us to look forward to our future in Heaven. We will never experience perfect or enduring fellowship with anyone in this world. But in Heaven, where there will be no more sin and death, there will be no more broken relationships. Recognizing these many beneficial aspects of loneliness is an important part of overcoming it.

Step 3: Get to Know God Better

The third step to overcoming loneliness is *to develop an intimate relationship with God.* For those who are not yet believers, this requires a new birth in Christ. We become sons of God only by realizing our need for a Savior, confessing our sins, repenting of them, and professing faith in Jesus Christ alone for salvation.

For those of us who are Christians, this requires practicing the presence of God. In other words, we need to actively seek to develop a deeper relationship with the Lord so that He is central to everything we think, say and do, every hour of every day. I know of a man who wanted to develop this type of relationship with God so much that he got a kitchen timer and set it for fifteen minutes. Every fifteen minutes that timer would "ding" and he would be reminded to think about God and to pray. He did this for several weeks, consciously directing his attention towards God every fifteen minutes of the day in order to develop a habit of thinking about God.

There are many other ways we can go about practicing the presence of God. Margaret Clarkson, a single woman, wrote a book called, *So You're Single.* In that book she wrote:

"My loneliness has driven me to seek and cultivate
Christ's companionship. My married friends had no

such gnawing need except in a general way. Without realizing it, they had been depending on one another for fellowship, and when that was lacking, they felt lost. I, never having known such companionship, constantly turned to God for fellowship, which enabled me to happily live alone anywhere."[9]

Later, she went on to describe how she turned to God and found companionship in Him. Whether we are married or unmarried, we all need to do this as well. We need to practice the presence of God.

Step 4: Put Off/Put On

The fourth step to overcoming loneliness is *to identify and eliminate the attitudes and actions that promote loneliness and then develop the attitudes and actions that promote good relationships*. There are many sinful attitudes and actions that can lead to loneliness–hostility, busyness, laziness, fear, perfectionism, self-centeredness, and others. If we wish to overcome loneliness, we need to properly deal with sinful attitudes and actions.

At the same time, however, we need to work at developing the attitudes and actions that promote deep and intimate relationships. The fruits of the Spirit are an excellent summary of these things: "...love, joy, peace, patience, kindness, goodness, faithfulness, gentleness, self-control" (Galatians 5:22-23). Any person who is full of these qualities is going to have a life rich in deep and meaningful relationships.

David's best friend Jonathan is an excellent example of someone who knew how to be a friend. 1 Samuel records the life of Jonathan and shows how he was committed to his friend, David, how he sacrificed for him, protected him, remained loyal to him even when it was difficult, and was even willing to lay down his own life for David. If we carefully and deliberately develop the friendship qualities evidenced in the life of Jonathan, we may be sure that we will have friends.

There are other passages in Scripture that teach us how to be a real friend. The one-another commands of the New Testament are good passages to study. For example, Romans 12:10 says, "Be devoted to one another in brotherly love..." People will naturally be drawn to us if they see that we are devoted to them, completely committed to them, and genuinely concerned about their welfare. On the other hand, people will be put off if they sense we are not really that interested in them.

There are many more commands like this. Romans 12:10 continues, "...give preference to one another in honor." In other words, we are to put other people ahead of ourselves. This means that we will be willing to sacrifice for them, we will encourage them, and we will look for ways to meet their needs. True friendships require this kind of life.

Later on in that same passage we are instructed to "be of the same mind toward one another" (Romans 12:16), and in Romans 14:13, "Therefore let us not judge one another anymore, but rather determine this–not to put an obstacle or a stumbling block in a brother's way." One of the greatest hindrances to deep friendship is a critical spirit. If we are the type of person who always complains, always condemns, and always finds fault, then we need to change. Instead, we should be genuinely concerned for others. One of the best antidotes for depression caused by loneliness is to reach out to others with the hand of friendship.

Along the same lines, Romans 15:7 says, "Therefore, accept one another, just as Christ also accepted us to the glory of God." We need to communicate to other people that we accept them. That does not mean that we condone or agree with everything they do, but rather that we receive and love them because Christ did the same for us. Christ accepted us by grace, not for anything that we did or did not do, and that is how we ought to accept other people as well.

Studying the "one-another" passages in Scripture will be very beneficial in helping us to better understand our responsibilities to other believers and the qualities that will produce meaningful relationships. It is my firm conviction, supported by numerous examples of people that I have counseled through severe loneliness, that those who struggle in this way are failing in some aspect of these one-another commands and qualities. And I am equally convinced that lonely people can develop deep and satisfying friendships when they put these things into practice.

Step 5: Putting it into Practice

How can we put these things into practice in our lives? First, as I already mentioned, we ought to do a careful and thorough study of all the one-another commands given in Scripture. One way to do this would be to get a concordance and use it to go through Scripture, looking for all the passages that talk about our responsibilities to other people. This could be part of a daily devotion time, and it would be helpful to write each of the commands down.

Second, we need to evaluate ourselves on each of the relationship responsibilities that we find in Scripture. A list should be made of the various commands and qualities and then ratings given on how we are doing, using the following criteria: "I always do this," "I frequently do this," "I sometimes do this," I seldom do this," or "I never do this." Any item on the list that is given a "sometimes," "seldom," or "never" needs improvement.

Third, we should think carefully and make a list of specific people with whom we will practice these things on a regular basis. For those of us who are married, our spouse and children should be first on the list. Then, the list can be expanded to include specific friends, other family members, neighbors, church members, etc. with whom we interact on a regular basis.

Fourth, make a list of at least thirty specific ways we will put a one-another command into practice with another person. For example, we might write something like, "I will serve John S. by helping him fix his car." Each item should be a specific idea of how we can best serve that person. Or, "I will encourage Mary B. by writing a note to let her know how much I appreciate her cheerfulness." Or, "I will live in harmony with Jan E. by allowing her to plan the program for the women's missionary meeting."

Fifth, we might keep a record for a period of seven to eight weeks in which we write down each day all the times and ways that we fulfilled the objectives on our list. Tracking our progress in this way will help us to be encouraged by what God is enabling us to do and will also motivate us to continue doing these things.

I am convinced that if we will follow this biblical plan for developing deep and intimate friendships, it will not be long before many of us can say, "On life's pathway I am seldom lonely." If we implement the biblical truths in this chapter, we can become people whose experience with loneliness becomes an experience of less loneliness. God has given us in the Scriptures all that we need for life and godliness. We have all the resources in God's Word we need to develop a deep and intimate relationship with God, and deep and intimate relationships with other people.

May God help us then to not merely hear what He has to say, but to walk in obedience, as James 1:25 exhorts us to do. May God help each of us to grow in our knowledge of His Word, and to change where we need to change. As we examine ourselves and seek to grow, God will give us the power and strength to glorify Him and to live full, satisfying, and meaningful lives.

QUESTIONS FOR DISCUSSION AND APPLICATION:

1. Do you agree with the statement that loneliness is a very common experience?

2. What biblical examples of loneliness are found in God's Word?

3. Do you know any really lonely people? Do you ever feel lonely?

4. What was meant by the statement that loneliness can be a very destructive experience? In what ways can this be true?

5. Do you agree with the statement that one of the causes of loneliness is a deficient relationship with God? Why is this true?

6. What is meant by the statement that one of the causes of loneliness is the transient nature of life?

7. One of the causes of loneliness is the nature of our responsibilities and commitments. How can this be true? Give examples.

8. What is meant by the statement that one of the causes of loneliness is our sins and our failures? How can this be true? Give examples.

9. It was stated that to solve the blues of loneliness we must accept the unavoidable. How is this possible?

10. One way to solve the blues of loneliness is to rejoice in the benefits of aloneness. What are some of the benefits of aloneness?

11. What is mean by the statement that to overcome the blues of loneliness we must practice the presence of God? How can we do this?

12. Another way to overcome loneliness is to practice the put off/put on dynamic. What must we put off and what must we put on to overcome the blues of loneliness?

13. Have you personally experienced a case of the blues of loneliness? Explain the specifics of the situations related to your case of the blues of loneliness.

14. What have you personally, or for the sake of helping others, learned from this chapter about the causes of loneliness that will be helpful in your own life or in your ministry to others?

15. Do the things presented in this chapter as the causes of loneliness make biblical sense? In other words, are they supported by Scripture?

Chapter 7
Questions and Answers About Depression

1. How do you keep a counselee from continually rehearsing their problems?

    You do what God did with Elijah and Jonah: You ask questions that will direct them. The kinds of questions that you ask will direct the conversation.

    I counseled a woman who constantly rehearsed her woes in our sessions together and at one point I said to her, "You are just exacerbating the situation by going over it again and again and again. Has that helped? Has that really resolved the problem? Temporarily, it may make you feel better to be able to say it aloud, but in reality you're hurting yourself when you do that. If I continue to allow you to do this, I'm hurting you."

    In that situation, it was so ingrained in her that she had a really hard time controlling herself. So I made up a little 3 x 5 card, with a picture of a CD player on it, and we agreed that every time she started to rehearse her woes, I would just hold up the card and say, "You're playing that same old song again." And that was a reminder to her that she should stop rehearsing her complaints.

    As a counselor, it's important to be a good listener, yet at the same time it's important to not allow a counselee to continually rehearse the same sorrows and woes again and again.

2. How does a person control or get rid of recurring or automatic thoughts?

    You get rid of automatic, sinful thoughts by making a habit of replacing them with godly thoughts. It's the put-off/put-on dynamic from Colossians 3:8-10 and elsewhere. If you know that you are stuck in a cycle of sinful thinking, you have to plan ahead in terms of what you are going to think about when those thoughts come. If you wait until the cycle starts to try to think of something else, it will be very difficult to think constructively. Do as Joseph did in Egypt when he prepared for the coming famine. He knew that seven years of plenty would be followed by seven years of want so he stored up for the later during the former.

In the same way, you need to think and plan types of things you will focus your mind on at a time when you are not in the midst of your sinful thoughts. It could be that you might find some Bible verses to meditate on, or a tape to listen to that has a sermon or other message on it, or some activity that will engage your mind so fully that it can't dwell on other things. Whatever legitimate activity works for you, do it, but prepare ahead.

I counseled a woman like this and she thought she would never break free of her automatic thoughts, but she did. She would wake up in the middle of the night with her mind racing through these sinful thoughts, and I helped her to plan ahead in terms of what she would do instead. Over a period of time she trained herself to think differently and broke out of that cycle from which she thought she would never be free. So it's a process, but it can be done. The Scripture teaches us to "… discipline yourself for the purpose of godliness" (1 Timothy 4:7), and this is an excellent example of what that means.

3. What is your approach to children who have been diagnosed with depression, especially those who may have come from a family in which there was a divorce?

     I believe that the underlying causes of depression are the same for children as they are for adults. I don't see any difference in terms of what the Word of God has to say about the nature of and solution to our problems for any person—young or old, man or woman, etc. I know that secular counselors disagree, but frankly, I'm not really all that concerned about what the world has to say about it. Each school of thought—the psycho-analysts, the behaviorists, the sociologists, the biologists—have a different view of the causes and development of depression.

I come to the problem of depression from the perspective of God's Word because I believe it contains everything that we need for life and godliness (2 Peter 1:3). In reference to children, it is often the case that children believe themselves to be "bad." They may have heard mom and dad arguing over them so they came to the conclusion that they are the cause of the divorce. They think perhaps if they had been more obedient, maybe mom and dad wouldn't be getting divorced. And so there is guilt—whether necessary or unnecessary. Though they haven't violated any of God's standards, they have replaced God's standards with some other standard so there is true, though unnecessary, guilt.

On the other hand, children may have unbiblical goals and values. They are sinners as well and when expectations or desires they value highly are not fulfilled, they can get very unhappy about it. I recall a couple who brought their son to me for counseling some time ago. This boy was only six or seven years old and had tried to commit suicide. When I saw him, he was very depressed, so I talked with him alone in our first session together. After that, however, I worked only with his parents because I believe that God has given parents to children to be their counselors. Ephesians 6:4 says, "Fathers, do not provoke your children to anger, but bring them up in the discipline and instruction of the Lord." The word translated "instruction" means "counsel."

I believe that parents should work to identify their children's problems and help them to solve those problems. As I worked with the parents on this, I discovered that the couple had some serious problems in their marriage and also lacked good parenting skills. I worked with them in terms of their personal lives, their maturity in Christ, their marriage relationship, and how they interacted with their son. As the parents' lives improved, the son improved as well. He started working harder and behaving better in school and I only saw him once more–at our last session together.

That is basically the approach that I like to take with children—counseling the parents to counsel their child. Now if the parents will not cooperate in that way, then I would agree to see just the child. But the child really needs to see good role models at home and to have the support and counsel of his parents in order to overcome his problems.

4. You have made several statements about counseling depressed people such as, "Use questions to gently challenge them to evaluate their expectations and convictions," and, "Be very patient with these people. Be slow to reprimand and when you do, it is usually best to do it in an oblique or indirect fashion." Understanding what Proverbs says about how it is the mark of a fool to be unable to receive a rebuke, to what extent are we breeding fools by reprimanding in only an oblique or indirect fashion?

> The principle I am using here is that we are to be "shrewd as serpents and innocent as doves" (Matthew 10:16). Or as Proverbs 12:18 says, "There is one who speaks rashly like the thrusts of a sword, but the tongue of the wise brings healing." In other words, speak in such a way that your listener will be able to hear what you are saying so as not to stir up a sinful response.

> Jesus did this many times by answering people with a question rather than a direct rebuke. It is possible to be direct but to do it in an indirect fashion. For example, when God questioned Jonah about his response to Nineveh's repentance, He asked Jonah, "Do you have good reason to be angry?" (Jonah 4:4). He could have said something like, "Jonah, I can give you ten good reasons why you shouldn't be angry about this!"

> Proverbs 15:2 says, "The tongue of the wise man makes knowledge acceptable..." So when we're counseling someone, we need to ask ourselves, "How can I best address this issue so that this person will listen to me and accept what I am saying?" I think that's the mark of wisdom. Evading an issue is one thing, but addressing an issue graciously and helpfully is another.

Depression and Other Problems

1. What association is there between anger and depression?

    There are several factors that contribute to the development
    of depression. In some cases, it's difficult to tell which is
    the chicken and which is the egg—whether a problem such
    as anger came first and then depression, or the other way
    around. Obviously, an angry person is not going to be a happy
    person; you cannot hold onto anger, bitterness, resentment
    or hostility and not experience unhappiness. On the other
    hand, it's certainly true that when a person is experiencing
    depression—even mild or moderate depression—it is much
    easier for them to become frustrated and for anger to spill over
    from that. As a counselor, data gathering is important for the
    purpose of discovering which came first, if possible. But anger
    is certainly a common component of depression.

2. What is the association between anxiety and depression, and how
    do you help someone with panic attacks, panic disorders, and
    other DSM labels?

    Again, depression often goes hand in hand with other
    problems. If you are a very anxious and worried person, you
    cannot be very joyful. And in some instances it really doesn't
    matter which is causing which because both need to be dealt
    with. If someone has a problem with anxiety, they need to be
    counseled in terms of their anxiety, panic, etc. The counselor
    should get them to think about how the Bible would have them
    deal with their panic so that they can experience more of the
    peace of God that passes all understanding.

    To do this, refer back to the section about the defeat of
    depression. I don't like to be simplistic in terms of my approach
    because I want people to understand that God does not just
    have a little to say about these things. He has quite a bit to
    say about them, and the tragedy is that we often write Him
    off so quickly. We think the Bible doesn't have the answers or
    insights that we need for these very common problems. The
    truth is that it does; we just haven't studied it enough.

3. How can Scripture be used to help people who are dealing with other "mental disorders" like obsessive-compulsive disorder?

It is important, whenever you are counseling someone like that, to gather a great deal of information in order to discover what theological issues may be involved in their problems. A wrong concept of God—not understanding justification by grace through faith—can contribute to these things. Fear of man or an inordinate desire to be a people-pleaser can be a part of it as well.

For example, people who constantly wash their hands may be struggling with a sense of guilt. They don't have freedom in Christ as Romans 8:1 says, "Therefore there is now no condemnation for those who are in Christ Jesus." A man I once counseled would drive out of the church parking lot and suddenly find himself frightened, "I think I hit someone as I left the parking lot." He would go to bed at night and think, "Did I lock the front door?" He would leave home in the morning and then wonder, "Did I turn the stove off? Is the house going to burn down?" If he bumped into someone accidentally in the street, he would think, "They probably think I want to sexually abuse them."

In all of these thoughts, he was focused on himself, not on what was pleasing to the Lord. So one of the things I did with him was to get him thinking about Romans 12:2, "And do not be conformed to this world, but be transformed by the renewing of your mind..." His mind was filled with the fear of man and he needed to fill his mind instead with the Word of God so that he could be God-centered rather than man-centered in his thoughts. Helping people to develop a right concept of God and true God-centeredness in their lives is very important.

Physical/Genetic Factors and Depression

1. Have you heard of the book *Sugar Blues*, and what are the nutritional factors in reference to depression?

I haven't heard of that particular book, but I've read other books that sound similar to it. A scientist by the name of Dr.

Feingold did a lot of research on food colorings and other such things and studied how they affected certain people. I think different substances do affect people differently. Since sugar, for example, stimulates some of the body's glands, some people experience a physically "high" effect from it. Feeding that high effect can lead to a sugar addiction. I have a friend who is very sensitive to caffeine. If he drinks a cup of coffee, he's climbing the walls for hours afterward. But I know other people who can drink cups of coffee and go to bed at night and sleep well. So caffeine affects people in different ways.

It is certainly possible that, due to their physiological make-up, some people are physically affected by certain substances in ways that other people are not. If you know that about yourself, you should stay away from that substance.

2. Is it wrong to refer to depression as a mental illness?

I do not refer to depression as a mental illness because I don't think the Bible does. What I mean by that is that the Bible does not refer to depression and other such problems (anxiety, for example) as being physical ailments. A mental illness is a disease of the brain—a tumor, an abscess, etc. It is something physiological. Any problem that is non-physical in nature should not, in my estimation, be termed a "disease" or "illness".

3. What evidence currently exists regarding a genetic tendency toward depression?

At this time there is much controversy on that subject. To my knowledge, nothing has yet been identified in a conclusive way. Dr. Bob Smith, a physician, explains that there is often a cause and effect link made between two things that have not been proven to be related. For example, one study has found that some depressed people have a certain physical deficiency that causes the depression.

Dr. Smith argues against this kind of thinking by using this illustration: Someone does some research and discovers that everyone who ate carrots in 1850 is now dead, so the conclusion is drawn that eating carrots caused their death. Therefore, don't eat carrots. Obviously, the fact that people ate carrots in 1850 has no connection with the fact that they are dead. While this illustration may be extreme, it shows the kind of poor thinking that often occurs in these types of studies. The fact that two problems coexist doesn't necessarily prove that the one causes the other.

To prove a causal relationship, you would have to examine a large number of people who had a particular genetic deficiency and find that they all experienced depression. You would also have to prove that there were not any other factors unique to that group of people that could be a part or cause of the problem. In other words, it is very difficult to definitively prove this kind of thing.

A real-life example of a study like this was done in La Jolla, CA, that sought to find some genetic basis for homosexuality. Scientists examined the brains of a number of people after death and discovered that certain parts of the brains of those who were homosexuals were smaller than the corresponding parts in people who were not homosexuals. The scientist who did the study admitted that it was inconclusive in terms of providing a genetic basis for homosexuality, but the media used the study to declare that a genetic basis for homosexuality had been found.

The problem with making such an assertion is that all of the homosexuals who died had AIDS, and who knows what AIDS does to the brain? The assumption was made that since part of the brain was smaller in some of the homosexuals, this was what caused the homosexuality. In order for that to be true, several other things would have to be also proven; in part that AIDS had not caused part of the brain to shrink in size, or that their homosexuality had not caused part of the brain to be smaller. Also, the study found that some of the brains of those who were not known to be homosexuals had the same brain characteristic as those who were.

So in reality the study proved nothing. And even if we suppose that eventually some genetic basis is found for depression, it only means that people with those genes have a predisposition to depression, not that they are unwilling and unwitting victims of it.

4. Are physiological problems ever hereditary? Can there literally be a chemical imbalance in the brain that has been inherited?

The problem with this diagnosis is that in most instances, scientists and doctors have offered this explanation—a chemical imbalance—because they have no other explanation and people are demanding one. When someone tells me they have been diagnosed with a chemical imbalance or something to that effect, I ask them what laboratory tests were done on them to make that analysis. In most cases, nothing was done. The doctors just ran out of options for explaining their problems.

Even if a doctor is able to prove some kind of chemical deficiency or other physical defect, that alone does not prove that the spiritual and emotional problems are a result of that. As stated previously, the fact that two things are present at the same time does not necessarily mean that one is causal; it just means they are both present at the same time. It may very well be as demonstrated in Dr. S. I. McMillen's book, *None of These Diseases*, that many physical problems may be caused by spiritual and emotional problems. In other words, the emotional and spiritual problems may be the chicken (the cause) rather than the egg (the result) of the problem.

5. Do you believe that a physical defect or deficiency (if found) that caused or contributed to depression could be a result of the curse?

First, no definitive link between a physical deficiency and depression has been proven, and there is much debate between scientists over the little evidence that has been found. But speaking hypothetically, I would say that if it were true, it could still never be used as an excuse for sinful behavior.

There is no sin in having a down mood—Jesus experienced great sadness in the Garden of Gethsemane and yet He did the will of the Father. The problem is, when the world seeks out these physical explanations for depression, it is often because they want an excuse for their sinful behavior. The Bible does not allow that, however. No matter how badly I may be feeling,

I can still do what God wants me to do. I do not have to let my feelings control me. When I have a bad headache, it may be easier to be nasty and irritable, but the Bible never allows me to use that as an excuse for acting or thinking sinfully.

In the end, it really doesn't matter whether a link is ever established between depression and the physical body because it will still never give us an excuse to sin.

6. You said that in a small percentage of cases where a person has a severely depressed mood, there may be a physiological component. How can that be diagnosed and what does it mean?

First, I am only saying that in a small percentage of cases, there is a definite physiological link to the mood disorder. For example, I am a diabetic and when my blood sugar gets out of control, I feel very sluggish and have a tendency towards feeling despondent. That physical problem with my blood sugar can be proven with a blood test, but again, it does not excuse any sinful behavior I may engage in because of the way that I feel.

Second, some doctors (like Dr. Bob Smith) argue that we should change the terms we use for these kinds of things to differentiate between what is known to be physically linked and what is not. So if someone has a hormonal imbalance due to an underactive thyroid problem, they are not diagnosed as having depression, but rather as having "hypothyroidism" or something like that.

7. Could you address the difference between a disorder and a disease as it relates to depression? And do you think it's fair to say that depression is a symptom of—in the majority of cases—a spiritual problem, and in the minority of cases, an actual disease?

First, I do not see depression as a disease. A disease is entirely physical and, in most cases, when someone has a disease, they are not responsible in any way for that disease occurring in their body. I don't believe the Bible puts depression in that category so I would never use that terminology in connection with depression.

Second, I would not say that depression is a disease or a symptom of a disease. If a certain mood is brought on by a physical ailment, then it should be called a symptom of that disease. But I don't think it should be called depression.

The Dynamics of Depression

1. Most, if not all, of the people in your example cases have had their focus primarily on themselves. Therefore, in the final analysis, are we not saying that the cause of depression is this inordinate emphasis on self?

    I think that a focus on self is certainly one of the things that occur in a depressed person. My discussion about the development of depression earlier in this book emphasizes the role that a preoccupation with self plays in depression.

2. Can you become severely depressed without knowing it?

    I suppose you could become severely depressed without being labeled as such, or calling it that yourself, but you can't become severely depressed without having some of the experiences that would characterize depression. A person may not call their experience "depression"—they may call it something else—but if it has all of the symptoms we have discussed, it is very likely depression. Ultimately, it really doesn't matter what we call it, it's what we understand and do about it that matters.

3. Do you believe that depression comes in stages? How do you view the progression of depression?

    Primarily, I think that whatever we practice we get better at, whether it's something good or bad. So someone who is in the habit of practicing the things that lead to depression will progressively become more deeply depressed. A person may be mildly depressed and then, because they fail to deal with it properly, may become moderately depressed. If they don't deal with that properly, they may become severely depressed.

Proverbs 17:14 illustrates this principle in terms of strife (or conflict). "The beginning of strife is like letting out water, so abandon the quarrel before it breaks out." In other words, the time to deal with a problem like strife is before it really gets started.

The same is true for depression. The time to nip depression is when it begins. When people become depressed, they often don't deal with the root things that are causing the depression. Instead they make a change in their circumstances–they go on vacation, or treat themselves to a shopping or eating spree. Sometimes they move to a new place. The bad mood is lifted temporarily, but they haven't dealt with the root cause. When something else happens, the depression comes right back to the surface because its real cause was never resolved.

For a while, we can divert ourselves from our problems by doing pleasant things, but after a while the pleasant things don't work the same way. It's much like medicine that someone takes to treat chronic pain. It works for a while but then eventually there comes a point where the pain becomes so bad that even the medicine doesn't help anymore. That's the kind of thing that often happens with people who struggle with depression.

4. Is there any truth in the concept of "seasonal" depression—feelings of lowness in the winter due to less sunlight?

If you're referring to depression as simply a mood, there are some experts who would say there is a correlation. However, I see depression as more than a mood. I see it in terms of behavior—the way you interact with other people and your circumstances. In other words, your responses to how you feel. It is certainly true that we all experience highs and lows in terms of our mood, which may be a result of something we ate the night before, the lack of sunlight, the weather, or any number of other things.

In Alaska where they experience long periods of time with little or no light, it is true that the rates of suicide are higher at those times. So from an external point of view, yes, circumstances can influence how we feel. What we do with how we feel, however, is up to us. We can choose to allow our feelings to control us and choose to act in unbiblical ways, or we can choose to glorify God regardless of how we feel.

The Role of Antidepressant Drugs

1. What is the role of antidepressant drugs in counseling?

   I am not a physician, so I cannot prescribe medication of any kind. However, many of the people that come to me want to get off an antidepressant drug. In many instances, they have endured a long period of trial and error—trying this drug and that at various dosages—and nothing seems to be working.

   When they come to me, I don't focus on the drugs. I focus on helping them to understand the issues I think are involved in the development of their depression and work on helping them to resolve those issues. If they ask me about the drugs they are taking, I suggest they ask their doctor if the drugs can be reduced or eliminated. They then take themselves off the drugs on their own under the supervision of a physician.

2. If someone is taking antidepressant medication and wants to stop, how exactly do you go about helping them do that?

   First, all counselors should have a *Physician's Desk Reference* which tells them the side-effects, the withdrawal symptoms, etc. of any drug a counselee may be taking. When working with a person who wants to get off the drugs, you would counsel them as to what to expect as they decrease or stop their dosage. You would tell them that they may or may not experience side-effects as they change their medication dosage, but it's important for them to be prepared for what could happen. As mentioned earlier, coming off the medicine or reducing the medicine should be done in connection with their physician so that the doctor can monitor their progress, etc. For most people with whom I have worked, it has not been a big problem because, at that point, they really do want to trust Christ and solve their problems biblically.

A woman I counseled some time ago had been diagnosed as manic-depressive and obsessive-compulsive. She was on Lithium when we started counseling, but she wanted to get off it. Eventually she did get off, although not because I told her or even suggested that she should. She began to deal with the challenges and stresses of life biblically and then went to her doctor and asked his help in getting off the Lithium. He gave her a warning and then reluctantly agreed. She came off the Lithium without any serious side effects and has been off it ever since. That woman took courses in biblical counseling and was hired as a counselor in a biblical counseling center and is doing wonderfully well today. At one time the doctors had told her that she would be on Lithium for the rest of her life.

3. How can we apply this teaching to people who are taking anti-depressant drugs such as Lithium, Prozac, etc.?

I counsel people according to a seven element process which is described in chapters 10-16 of the book, *Introduction to Biblical Counseling.*[10] I won't try to go through that process in detail right now, but I will highlight a few things.

First, I talk to the person about their view of the authority of Scripture. I explain that God knows far more about why we have problems and what to do about them than anyone else and I ask them if they are willing to look at what the Scripture has to say. If they say, "Yes," then I continue by working through the development and dynamics of depression from a biblical perspective with them. I challenge them to commit themselves to solving their problem God's way.

I do not have a medical degree, and if someone I am counseling is on some kind of medication, it would be illegal for me to either prescribe or de-prescribe those meds. I don't tell people to take drugs or stop taking them. In fact, I sometimes don't discuss the drug issue at all unless or until they bring it up, or if some of the symptoms they are experiencing are similar to the ones mentioned as side effects of the kind of drugs they are taking. I don't allow the drugs to become the focus of the counseling. If any of the symptoms may possibly be side effects of the drugs they are taking, I don't play physician. Rather, I send them to the physician to discuss their symptoms and ask for his counsel. Quite honestly, most of the people with whom I work who are on drugs want to get off them. When they ask me about it, I suggest they talk to their doctor about reducing or stopping the medication. In most cases, doctors have been very willing to cooperate because many of them realize that pills aren't the answer either.

Suicide and Depression

1. In nursing school, I was taught that if a person talks about suicide or being depressed, we should take it very seriously because it is a key factor in terms of the possibility of suicide. In light of what you have been teaching, are there other things that need to be taken into consideration as well?

If anyone talks about committing suicide, I think we ought to take it seriously. There are many different motives for people to say they are thinking about committing suicide. Sometimes it may be because they want to get someone else's attention and they can't think of anything more serious than for them to threaten suicide.

But how do you distinguish between someone who is just playing games and someone who is really serious? Personally, I just take everyone who says something like that seriously. For example, there have been instances when a woman was expecting her husband home at a certain time, so she took an overdose of drugs a few minutes before he was due home, hoping that he would find her in that state but still alive. She hoped he would realize how unhappy she was and be willing to make some changes. But when the husband had a flat tire on the way home and didn't arrive until much later, his wife was already dead.

I've worked with people who have made numerous attempts at suicide but have seemingly not been able to pull it off. They were filled with self-pity and they wanted to be the center of attention. I take any "threat" seriously, though there are many things we need to take into account when working with people–emotional, cognitive, motivational, behavioral, social, and historical aspects.

2. What would be the reason for suicide being the second leading cause of death among college students?

> Suicide is a leading cause of death for that age group and occurs most frequently during exam time for college students. Suicide may be higher than other causes of death because students feel pressured to excel in school and may not be living up to the standard they have set for themselves. At exam time, many students survive on minimal sleep and do all sorts of crazy things as a result. Also, they may feel as if there is no purpose in life, which is not surprising based on what they are being taught at secular schools. The existentialism, pessimism, negativism, and lack of absolute standards that are presented in these ungodly schools almost makes one wonder why more unsaved young people don't try to take their lives. There is no meaning in life apart from Jesus Christ and nothing makes sense without Him.

Theology and Depression

1. What differences are there between depression in the Old Testament and depression in the New Testament—how it develops, etc.?

> I don't believe there is any difference. Though I have used many examples from the Old Testament, there are some to be found in the New Testament as well: the disciples on the Emmaus road, the experience of Judas Iscariot, and the experience Paul describes in 2 Corinthians 4 are just a few examples. All aspects of depression are very much the same in the Bible. The experiences of God's people in the Old Testament who experienced depression are, just like the "heroes of the faith" in Hebrews 11, a model and example for us.
>
> It is my personal theological conviction that you cannot be saved or sanctified without the work of the Holy Spirit. David prayed in Psalm 51:11, "...do not take Your Holy Spirit from me." It is impossible to obey God without the Holy Spirit. We have a lot more understanding about the ministry of the Holy Spirit in the New Testament, but the Spirit is always necessary for salvation.

2. You have indicated that you don't believe Satan can get into our thoughts. If that is true, how do we account for our minds wandering during Bible reading, prayer, and even church?

> Frankly, I don't need any help from Satan to do that. My indwelling sin is very capable of doing that by itself. No, I don't believe that Satan can make me sin, but Scripture indicates that until we get to Heaven, we will struggle with our "old man"—the indwelling sin that used to be our master.
>
> In looking at the Scripture, we see that Paul never blamed someone's thoughts or deeds on the devil. He always held people accountable for their actions. He pointed out their sin and told them to repent of it and walk in obedience. In 1 Corinthians 3:1-3 he said, "And I, brethren, could not speak to you as to spiritual men, but as to men of flesh, as to infants in Christ. I gave you milk to drink, not solid food; for you were not yet able to receive it. Indeed, even now you are not yet able, for you are still fleshly. For since there is jealousy and strife among you, are you not fleshly, and are you not walking like mere men?" The problem is our flesh—the remnants of our sinful nature, habit patterns developed in our pre-Christian days—not Satan causing us to sin.

3. You have said much about reading the Psalms, and Scripture commands us to use Psalms in personal and corporate worship (Ephesians 5:19 and Colossians 3:16). Do you think Christians should seek to incorporate the Psalms more in their daily devotions? And do you agree that reading them can help someone with "the blues"?

> I think that's an excellent idea. All Scripture is given by the inspiration of God and is helpful to us. The Psalms are especially meaningful because, for the most part, they are about man speaking to God. And they are very instructive because they are inspired in terms of what they speak about to God.
>
> The book of Psalms reflects upon the richest collection of life's experiences in all Scripture. The honesty of emotion runs the gamut of godly praise and adoration to the depths of

despair. We find solace, comfort and joy in those pages. In the end, the lesson in the Psalms is that we conquer depression and loneliness by means of faith in the Living God.

4. As a biblical counselor, how do you—or should you—integrate various theories of secular thought into your counseling?

I don't. I look to the Scriptures alone because although there may be some secular theories that are illustrative of Scriptural principles, the Word of God is the only sufficient source of wisdom to deal with our problems.

I have no problem with scientific research psychology, where the goal is simply to observe and record behavior. For example, secular scientists are funded to do studies on what happens when people don't get enough sleep. They have found that many cognitive functions suffer when people are deprived of sleep, which simply reinforces or illustrates what the Bible already says about the importance of taking care of our bodies.

My primary source is always the Word of God. If I would use secular psychology at all, it would be to simply illustrate what I know from God's Word to be true, rather than as a source of truth itself. Clinical psychology, on the other hand, is counseling, not research. It's not scientific; if anything, it's theology, but bad theology because it's unbiblical.

Chapter 8
Additional Notes for the Counselor

It is my desire, in writing this book, to teach not just those who are struggling with depression on their own but also to instruct those who wish to counsel people with depression. In this chapter I have included some additional notes on useful techniques for counseling, important principles to keep in mind about counseling depressed people, and resource material for homework assignments for the counselee. For readers who are not counselors, I encourage you to read on and counsel yourselves as we noted in the lives of Asaph, Jeremiah, and David.

When working with a depressed person who has come for counseling, it is important to use questions to discover three things: one, the level of their experience of depression (mild, moderate, or severe); two, the specific nature of what is facilitating their depression (unresolved sin, unbiblical responses to difficulty, unbiblical values and expectations, or a physiological disorder); and three, what they have done so far to deal with their depression. This information is critical to being able to correctly and adequately address the counselee's problem.

From the beginning, it is important to determine the general mindset of a depressed person. Depressed people are so often entangled in their mental anguish that they have become virtually immobile and unable to deal with their top priority problems. In general, they are so absorbed in themselves that they talk about their problems constantly but never do anything about it. The counselor needs to remind the depressed person that: "When there are many words, transgression is unavoidable, but he who restrains his lips is wise" (Proverbs 10:19). Rehearsing and rehashing problems leads only to sin, not solutions.

They are also very feeling-oriented. In other words, they view the world and their circumstances through the subjective lens of their emotions–how things make them feel–and allow their feelings to have control over them. They are usually convinced that their situation is unique–that no one else in the world is as miserable as they or can understand the depth of their troubles.

When questioning the counselee, the counselor should first seek to determine the presentation problem. In other words, what is the counselee's understanding of their problem? How do they feel? For example: "I'm tired all the time. I cry a lot. I never get anything done and my friends just don't understand me." These statements may be the counselee's perception of the cause of their problems, but it is important for the counselor to understand this for what it really is: the effect. "A plan in the heart of a man is like deep water, but a man of understanding draws it out" (Proverbs 20:5).

Next, the counselor should seek to find out what the performance problem is. In other words, what specific thoughts and actions are producing these feelings? For example: "I've stopped doing chores around the house. I rarely go out anymore. I avoid talking to or being with my friends." From these statements the counselor can see that because their performance is not right (they aren't doing things they should be doing), their feelings are not right either.

The counselor should work to identify the pre-conditioning aspect. Is there unresolved sin in their life? Are they responding unbiblically to a difficult circumstance? Do they have unbiblical expectations, desires, etc.? How far back does the problem extend? What habits have been formed that make it easy for them to respond as they do now? Does it seem likely that the depression is being caused by a physical problem rather than a spiritual one? (If so, see "Physical Problems and their Relationship to Depression" later on in this chapter.)

As the counseling proceeds, the counselor must always be careful to minister to the counselee in a holistic way: physically, personally, theologically, cognitively, relationally, and motivationally. The counselee should be strongly encouraged to adopt a long-distance view of the process of overcoming depression. The changes that will need to be made in their lives must be seen as an on-going process, not an instant fix.

Because of the intensity of their struggle, severely depressed people often want quick results. When they don't get them, they are inclined to stop trying. They quickly lose confidence in the Lord and in the power of His Word because they have unrealistic expectations of what is involved in overcoming depression. As a result, they may look for unbiblical–and ultimately ineffective–ways to solve their problem, as the Israelites did, "For My people have committed two evils: they have forsaken Me, the fountain of living waters, to hew for themselves cisterns, broken cisterns that can hold no water" (Jeremiah 2:13).

The following diagrams depict the wholistic approach that should be used when dealing with the problem of depression. Diagram 1 depicts some of the various areas of a person's life that must be dealt with in the process of overcoming depression.

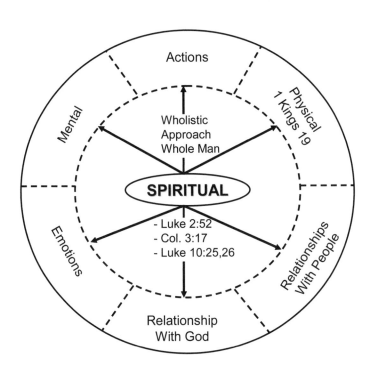

Diagram 2 demonstrates the reason why attention must be devoted to the various aspects of a person's life in the process of overcoming depression. The reason as illustrated by this diagram is that every area is being influenced by every other aspect of a person's life. I call this diagram the Interpersonal Dynamics of Influence and it is intended to portray this point. This fact makes it necessary to address and promote biblical obedience in a holistic way, which means that to overcome depression we must deal with all the important areas, not just one aspect of a person's life.

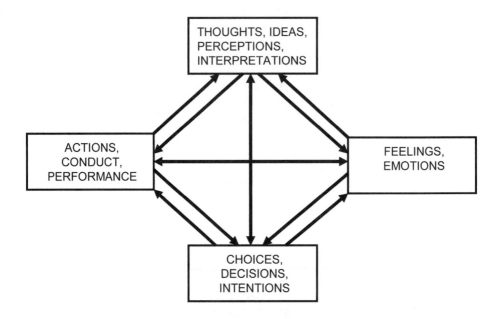

INTERPERSONAL DYNAMICS OF INFLUENCE

At this point, as we emphasize the importance of using a holistic approach in dealing with the problem of depression, I will include some suggestions that may be helpful for direction in using the holistic approach during counseling sessions or as homework assignments

Dealing with the Physical Area of the Person's Life

1. If the counselee has a number of factors that may indicate a physical component, discuss with them the importance of seeing a physician and undergoing a thorough physical exam.

2. Prescribe and encourage appropriate physical activity and/or exercise if that is something they are not doing presently.

3. Assess their diet and give them information for improvement or consult with a dietitian for further help.

4. Discuss with them any sleep difficulties they may be experiencing and the importance of regular sleep. Discuss appropriate relaxation and breathing exercises.

5. Provide them with information about medications, coffee, tea, and other stimulants or depressants that may be affecting them physically.

6. Encourage them to seek medical help for any physical problems– diseases, infirmities, etc.

   (Check the index and read what Dr. Robert writes about the physical aspects of a depressed mood in *The Christian Counselor's Medical Desk Reference.*)[11]

Dealing with the Theological Area of the Person's Life

1. Minister appropriate biblical hope to the counselee in frequent and massive doses.

2. Teach them a biblical perspective on the process of change and the importance of perseverance and endurance.

3. Show them you are there to do much more than simply listen to their problems and give them sympathy. Make sure they understand that God has answers to their problems and that you intend to challenge and encourage them with those answers.

4. Explore their concept of God and provide accurate, biblical insight about God in relevant ways.

5. Help them to formulate a biblical perspective on hardship, pain, and suffering.

6. Gently and humbly help them to see their circumstances and situation from a biblical perspective.

7. Address the root issues, as confirmed by sufficient data, of their depression. Help them to compare their thoughts, beliefs, values, interpretations and desires with Scripture. Judiciously explain how their thoughts, beliefs, etc., may be in conflict with Scripture and explain how they can change their thinking to bring it in line with Scripture.

8. Enlarge their concept of God's power, wisdom, mercy, and love towards them.

9. Give them relevant and helpful assignments to reinforce biblical concepts:

   a. Chapters from *Spiritual Depression: Its Causes and Cure*, by Martin-Lloyd Jones.

   b. *Knowing God*, by J. I. Packer.

   c. Bible book studies or topic studies (concordance or prepared) on God's grace, love, faithfulness, etc., and how it applies to their problem.

   d. *Trusting God*, by Jerry Bridges.

   e. *True Success and How to Attain It*, by Wayne Mack.

   f. *Down, But Not Out*, by Wayne Mack.

   g. *Anger and Stress Management God's Way*, by Wayne Mack.

   h. *God's Solutions to Life's Problems*, by Wayne and Joshua Mack.

   i. *The Fear Factor*, by Wayne and Joshua Mack.

   j. *A Fight to the Death*, by Wayne and Joshua Mack.

   k. *A Christian Growth and Discipleship Manual*, by Wayne Mack and Wayne Johnston.

   l. *Humility: A Forgotten Virtue*, by Wayne and Joshua Mack.

   m. *Theology of Christian Counseling*, by Jay Adams.

   n. *Christ and Your Problems*, by Jay Adams.

   o. *The Christian Counselor's Manual*, by Jay Adams.

Dealing with the Cognitive Area of the Person's Life

1. Use questions to gently challenge depressed persons to evaluate their interpretations, beliefs, expectations, and convictions.

2. Use vivid (picturesque, gripping) illustrations to drive home truth.

3. Teach them that progress and change will be a process involving setbacks and easy discouragement on their part.

4. Identify blame-shifting, rationalization, and irresponsibility that may facilitate and perpetuate depression.

5. Help them to identify and learn from previous positive or negative experiences that may be useful to them at the present time.

6. Help them to understand that emotions are connected to our thoughts, beliefs, values, interpretations, desires, and our personal evaluation of our behavior and circumstances.

7. Teach them to talk to themselves rather than listen to themselves, to ask questions of themselves, and to become aware of unbiblical assumptions, beliefs, and self-talk. Teach them to challenge and replace those things with biblical beliefs and self-talk. For example: "I can't do it," can be replaced with, "I haven't yet learned how, but with God's help I can do anything He wants for me." "I'm no good," can be replaced with, "I have Christ's righteousness."

8. Teach them to adopt and practice the ABC (Adversity Builds Character) view of their experience.

9. Have them start a journal where they record all the high and low points in their life and what made them high or low points.

10. If the counselee has been to other counselors in the past, write to those counselors (with the counselee's permission) and get the counselor's report of their insights and understanding of the counselee and their problems.

11. Have them keep a journal in which they answer the following questions on a daily basis:

- What events or circumstances (e.g. failures, criticisms, threats, etc.) am I experiencing that bring pressure on me at this time?

- What are my thoughts about these circumstances?

- What am I tempted to do or say in response to these circumstances?

- What feelings or emotions am I experiencing in response to these circumstances?

- What do I want that I am not getting? And what am I getting that I do not want? What desires of mine are being thwarted at this time?

- What is God's perspective–His truth–about the situation? What are His promises, instructions, and exhortations that apply to my situation? What would God want me to be thinking about the situation? What biblical truths apply to my situation?

- What desires would God want me to have at this time? What should I be wanting most of all? What would God say I should be most concerned about in this situation? What desires/motives should be driving and ruling me at this time?

- What actions or words would be pleasing to God?

- What will be my way of deliverance from the temptations that I am experiencing at this time?

- What will I choose to think, desire, do and say at this time?

12. Have them do a study on our resources in Christ found in *A Christian Growth and Discipleship Manual* by Wayne Mack and Wayne Johnston. Other hope-giving assignments are found in this book also.

13. Have them study and memorize Bible verses that present the biblical perspective on the unbiblical thoughts, desires, actions, etc., with which they have been struggling.

Dealing with the Relational Area of the Person's Life

1. Encourage the depressed person to develop appropriate, godly social relationships and, if possible, help to facilitate this in their life.

2. Have them do relevant studies from *Homework Manual, Vol. 1*, by Wayne Mack (loneliness, making friends), and *A Christian Growth and Discipleship Manual*, by Wayne Mack and Wayne Johnston. Numerous assignments are found in this book dealing with relational issues.

3. Give them appropriate material on developing godly social relationships (tapes, books, etc.).

4. Have them do a study on the "one-another" commands in Scripture.

5. Have them do a study of interpersonal relations from Proverbs or other passages, or a Bible study on fellowship or friendship.

6. Have them keep a meaningful contact journal.

7. Have them read *You Can Overcome Interpersonal Conflicts*, by Wayne Mack.

8. Have them read *The Crisis of Caring*, by Jerry Bridges.

9. Have them read *How to Help People in Conflict*, by Jay Adams.

10. Have them read *The Peacemaker*, by Ken Sande.

Dealing with the Motivational Area of the Person's Life

1. Encourage meaningful activity that is not overwhelming to the depressed person, and help them develop specific plans for their activities (breaking them down into manageable parts as necessary).

2. Provide them with appropriate and gentle challenges to fulfill their God-given responsibilities by breaking those responsibilities down into manageable parts. Help them develop a realistic plan for fulfilling their responsibilities.

3. Encourage them to have a God-centered hope, not hope that is centered in other people, circumstances, or their own abilities.

4. Avoid minimizing their thoughts of hostility, guilt, helplessness, etc., so that they do not feel misunderstood or patronized.

5. Help them acknowledge their pain and wait patiently for change in their life. Teach them that waiting hopefully does not mean doing nothing; rather, it means depending, expecting, enduring, and obeying. Teach them to stop looking for instant happiness.

6. Have them make a list of all the benefits that will result from changing, and all the misery and disadvantages of not changing. Have them make a list of biblical reasons for believing they can change.

7. Have them do a Bible study on the promises of God, hope, God's purpose for living, or God's purposes for trials and suffering.

8. Have them write out a statement of commitment to persevere in working on change.

Suggestions for homework assignments for helping a person whose depression is caused mainly by unresolved sin:

1. Read through the book, *True Success and How to Attain It*. The second half of this book focuses on God's forgiveness.

2. Do a Bible study of verses on repentance.

3. Do a Bible study of verses on forgiveness.

4. Do a Bible study on Psalms 32, 38, and 51.

5. Make a list of the consequences of sin and the benefits of obedience.

6. Read *Transforming Grace*, by Jerry Bridges.

7. Read *Disciplines of Grace*, by Jerry Bridges.

8. Read *Don't Waste Your Life*, by John Piper.

9. Read the book, *A Fight to the Death*, by Wayne Mack. This book discusses why sin is serious and how to put it to death.

10. Read *The Pilgrim's Progress*, by John Bunyan.

Suggestions for Understanding and Identifying the Presence of Physical Problems and Their Relationship to Depression

I mentioned briefly in previous chapters that, in a minority of cases, a depressed mood may be connected to a physical or organic problem rather than a spiritual one. For example, a depressed mood may be facilitated by physical problems such as sleep loss, a reaction to medications, a vitamin deficiency, poor diet, metabolic disease (diabetes, epilepsy, anemia, etc.), or glandular disease (hypothyroidism, etc.) Again I encourage you to read what Dr. Robert Smith has to say about the physical component of a depressed mood in *The Christian Counselor's Medical Desk Reference*. I am not a physician. Therefore I encourage you to research, as I did, what scientists like Dr. Smith and other physicians who are biblical counselors have to say about the physical components of some of the blues that people experience. Every issue of *The Journal of Modern Ministry* has a section written by godly physicians on biblical and scientific aspects of various physical problems. I also recommend a book written by Dr. S. I. McMillen titled, *None of These Diseases*. This book deals with the physical problems often related to unbiblical responses to the problems of life.

When assessing a person's depressed mood, it is important to be aware of this possibility and to ask questions that will help to uncover symptoms that may indicate such a problem. If a physical problem is suspected, the person should be strongly urged to undergo a thorough physical exam. The following questions are a result of the information I have gleaned from reading and listening to the presentations of several physicians on this subject. It should be noted that several positive responses to these questions are merely suggestive of a physical problem, not a definitive diagnosis of it. If a physical problem is indeed diagnosed by a medical doctor, the problem should then be identified by its disease nomenclature, not the term "depression."

QUESTIONS FOR THE COUNSELOR:

1. Has there been a serious impairment of the person's intellectual abilities?

2. Was the onset of the depression extremely sudden (severe depression occurring with no previous incidence)?

3. Did the depressed mood occur when there were no significant traumatic life events or flagrant violations of the person's personal standards that were closely related in time to the development of depression?

4. Does the individual have a track record of being a relatively secure, stable, confident, well-adjusted, realistic person?

5. Has the depressed person been a chronic blame-shifter or excuse-maker?

6. Are the person's somatic complaints few in number, specific, and continuous in nature?

7. Does the depressed person have a history of illusory somatic complaints?

8. Is the depressed person subject to sensory and non-persecutory, accusatory hallucinations?

9. Is the person delusional in an extreme and inexplicable way (not simply due to a lack of communication or misperception)?

10. Is the depressed person advanced in age?

11. Is the depressed person functioning biblically and really trying to act and think in a godly way?

12. Is the depressed person taking prescription, over-the-counter, or illegal drugs that have a depressant side-effect?

CASE STUDY FOR DISCUSSION AND APPLICATION

Your friend, Jim, tells you he is really depressed. You had an idea that something was wrong, but now it's out in the open. Jim is forty-five years old and has a wife and three children. He has been employed as a school teacher since he graduated from college twenty-three years ago. He claims to be a Christian and attends church regularly. In the past, he served in various capacities in the church–singing in choir, working with Boy's Brigade, teaching Sunday School, and serving as a deacon. Presently, he is not involved in any official service ministry of the church.

Jim says to you, "I'm really down. It's like a big empty feeling. Nothing seems important anymore. Almost everything has lost its meaning...teaching, my marriage, church activities, my sex life. I guess I still care about the children, but even there I feel kind of 'blah.' I can't seem to work up enthusiasm for anything anymore. I feel lousy most of the time. I can't remember the last time I felt good. I just can't do many of the things I used to be able to do. Sometimes I wonder why I should go on living. Why not end it all? God doesn't seem to care about me and nobody would really miss me if I were gone.'"

QUESTIONS TO DISCUSS:

1. Using the three categories of depression (mild, moderate, severe) as an evaluative tool, how depressed do you think Jim is and why do you think that?

2. What questions would you like to ask Jim about his depression? What other information would you like to know?

3. What might be the underlying cause(s) of Jim's depression?

4. What effects do you know or think depression is having on Jim's life?

5. What counsel would you give to Jim for dealing with his problem of depression?

Notes

1   *The Christian Counselor's Medical Desk Reference*, Timeless Texts.
2   Ibid.
3   Boice, James.
4   Ibid.
5   Krummacher, F.W., *Elijah*, Zondervan, Grand Rapids, pp 105-108.
6   Bunyan, John, *The Pilgrim's Progress*, Barry Horner, Ed. (North Brunswick, NJ), 1997.
7   Smith, Robert, M.D., *Journal of Pastoral Counseling*, Vol. 1, No. 1, pages 85-87.
8   MacArthur, John, *The Glory of Heaven*, pages 115-146.
9   Clarkson, Margaret, *So You're Single*.
10 Timeless Texts.
11 Ibid, Timeless Texts.

I conclude this book with a poem written by a friend of mine who spent a long time in the dark valley of depression, but now has a new and godly perspective on her depressive experience. I include this poem because it not only portrays how a depressed person is thinking and feeling while in the depths of depression, but also because in a beautiful and meaningful way it describes the hope and victory that comes when a person adopts a biblical perspective on the potentially depressing, unpleasant, and unwanted circumstances of life.

And Winter Came
By Joan Bob

I was not prepared for the winter winds that chill the bone,
With the desperate sense of being alone.
Alone except for Christ, my Rock, my strength, my sword,
My hope, my joy, my Lord.

Winter came, grace seemed to fail;
I suffered snow and ice and hail.
Relentless was the terrible pain;
I longed for gentle, warming rain.

The winds cut through my very soul,
And Christ alone could make me whole.
But only in His time, He said;
I wished and prayed that I were dead.

The days went by, then weeks, then years;
At times I thought I'd drown in tears.
Relentless still the pain I felt;
Yet always at His feet I knelt.

My question o'er and o'er was, "Why?"
"Because of love," was His reply.
I look back and now I see:
He sculpted, chiseled, molded me.

And if at times I ask Him, "Why?"
"Because I love you," He'll reply.
Today I have those warming rains,
The ones that wash away my pains.

The winds may come that chill the bone,
But now I know I'm not alone.
I trusted Him and sought His face,
And through the melted snow came grace.

(Used by permission)

Strengthening Ministries International

Strengthening Ministries International exists to provide training and resources to strengthen you and your church. We as individuals and as a ministry exist to glorify God by doing what Luke tells us Paul and his associates did in Acts 14:21 and 22. Luke tells us that Paul and his associates went about preaching the Gospel, making disciples, strengthening the souls of those disciples, and encouraging them to continue in the faith.

Like Paul we are dedicated to using whatever gifts and abilities, whatever training and experience, whatever resources and opportunities we have to strengthen individual Christians and churches in their commitment to Christ and in their ministries for Christ.

And like Paul, we are attempting to strengthen the church and individual Christians in a variety of ways. Fulfilling our ministry involves conducting seminars and conferences all over the United States and in many foreign countries. It includes writing and distributing books and booklets, and developing and distributing audio and videotapes on numerous biblical/theological/Christian life/counseling subjects.

Fulfilling our purpose for existence, as described in Acts 14:21,22, also includes developing and sustaining our website. On this website you will find fuller descriptions of the various aspects of our ministry as well as instructions about how to order materials. You may also contact us at P.O. Box 249, Center Valley, PA 18034.

Strengthening Ministries International
Resource Administrator: Charles Busby
P.O. Box 1656
Lacombe, LA 70445-1656
Phone: 985-882-3342 (Faxes can be received if you call this number first)
email: webmaster@mackministries.org